The Psychiatry *of* AIDS

The
Psychiatry
of AIDS

A Guide to Diagnosis and Treatment

Glenn J. Treisman, M.D., Ph.D.
and
Andrew F. Angelino, M.D.

Department of Psychiatry and Behavioral Sciences
The Johns Hopkins School of Medicine
Baltimore, Maryland

Foreword by John G. Bartlett, M.D.

The Johns Hopkins University Press
Baltimore and London

Drug dosage: The authors and publisher have exerted every effort to ensure that the selection and dosage of drugs discussed in this text accord with recommendations and practice at the time of publication. However, in view of ongoing research, changes in governmental regulations, and the constant flow of information relating to drug therapy and drug reactions, the reader is urged to check the package insert of each drug for any change in indications and dosage and for warnings and precautions. This is particularly important when the recommended agent is a new and/or infrequently used drug.

© 2004 The Johns Hopkins University Press

All rights reserved. Published 2004
Printed in the United States of America on acid-free paper
9 8 7 6 5 4 3 2

The Johns Hopkins University Press
2715 North Charles Street
Baltimore, Maryland 21218-4363
www.press.jhu.edu

Library of Congress Cataloging-in-Publication Data
Treisman, Glenn J., 1956–
    The psychiatry of AIDS : a guide to diagnosis and treatment / Glenn J. Treisman and Andrew F. Angelino ; foreword by John G. Bartlett.
        p. ; cm.
    Includes bibliographical references and index.
    ISBN 0-8018-7970-1 (hardcover : alk. paper) — ISBN 0-8018-8006-8 (pbk. : alk. paper)
    1. AIDS (Disease)—Patients—Mental health. 2. AIDS (Disease)—Psychological aspects.
        [DNLM: 1. HIV Infections—complications. 2. Case Reports. 3. HIV Infections—psychology. 4. Mental Disorders—etiology. 5. Mental Disorders—therapy. 6. Psychotherapy—methods. WC 503.5 T787p 2004]
I. Angelino, Andrew F. II. Title.
        RC606.6.T74 2004
        362.196'9792—dc22   2004004602

A catalog record for this book is available from the British Library.

For our patients, our wives, and our children

Contents

Foreword

Dr. Glenn Treisman has led the Psychiatric Services for the Johns Hopkins HIV/AIDS Care Program for more than a dozen years. Dr. Treisman is an expert in the skills of communication, as shown in his many lectures to HIV care providers, where he invariably scores the highest evaluations at any conference. He is one of the few speakers who provide analyses that actually change systems. His broad experience in psychiatry and AIDS and the gift of communication come together in this book in grand fashion.

The book is of particular importance for psychiatrists who need more information about AIDS and for HIV care providers who need more information about why their patients do what they do. Dr. Treisman and coauthor Dr. Andrew Angelino describe this as a "book of hope." The authors are from the Paul McHugh school, which has a tradition of profundity and an unshakable belief in the organic causality of selected conditions such as major depression, schizophrenia, and HIV dementia. It also acknowledges that much of what we see in our patients is situational—that is, a behavioral response to life circumstances, something that applies to everyone but which prompts different responses. Thus, some individuals have problems with life situations because they are organically impaired, some make bad decisions, and some respond in a way that is absolutely rational but reflects devastating life circumstances. All can be helped.

The psychiatric implications of HIV infection are immense, possibly more important in this disease than in almost any other. The authors work in the Moore Clinic, which has served about 5,000 HIV-infected patients from diverse populations, but most represent an urban population of economically disadvantaged patients, which reflects the mainstream HIV infection as we see it in this and most urban areas. About 25 percent have a major mental illness and a majority have life situations that merit psychiatric intervention. The main goals in the mental health care they receive from Dr. Treisman, Dr. Angelino, and their team are to improve the quality of life, to increase engagement in medical care (including adherence to HAART), and to modify behavior to reduce the probability of transmission. Few diseases exist in which all three components are so crucial in terms of outcome, survival, and epidemiology. These are the goals of their program and this book. It is interesting to review other books and sections of major textbooks dealing with HIV infection. Most divide the contents by various categories using a systems approach, a pathogen approach, or the stage of disease, but few have substantial material devoted to mental health except possibly the extreme conditions. Nevertheless, for many of us this may be one of the most important specialty areas.

An important component of this book is the practical information provided. Seven patient presentations are included—cases that will be immediately familiar to the reader with any experience in treating HIV. They are the patients we see every day and the situations we struggle with. The recommendations are presented with great clarity, including the tests to do, the medicines to give, and the expectations for outcome. Important information dealing with the convergence of mental health and HIV care is provided in tabular form, including drugs, doses, and drug interactions. In the era of polypharmacy for the HIV-infected patient, these are data that are critical for the routine management of these patients.

A particularly significant aspect of this book is the diversity of topics covered. Along with a discussion of the major psychiatric illnesses associated with HIV infection, there is a substantial section on substance abuse and sexual disorders. Also covered are health care provider burnout, therapeutic nihilism, and very practical guidance in the integration of psychiatric and HIV care. In this truly comprehensive text, the reader will find practical material based on the authors' long and continuing experience.

This is a good read for both HIV care providers and mental health professionals, with good synthesis, good advice, and good humor.

John G. Bartlett, M.D.
Stanhope Professor of Medicine and
Chief, Division of Infectious Diseases
Department of Medicine
Johns Hopkins University

Preface

This is a book of hope. It is a tribute to people who have changed their lives, worked toward good, and tried to be better. The patients mentioned in this book are a few of the hundreds we have treated who have gone on to live their lives in better ways. Although many of our patients died in the early 1990s, a time of terrible losses in this epidemic, this is a book about life, not about death. It is a tribute to the hope that comes from making something and doing something instead of giving up.

I have worked in the world of HIV care for 14 years and have recruited intelligent and committed doctors, nurses, psychologists, and therapists to help me. The work in this book is as much theirs as mine. Dr. Constantine Lyketsos, already a formidable psychiatric researcher and clinician who cares for patients with neuropsychiatric disorders, joined me almost immediately despite many more attractive and easier options. Dr. Marc Fishman, one of the brightest substance abuse psychiatry specialists I have known, also joined our incipient group. I was truly fortunate to be joined by Dr. Heidi Hutton, clinical psychologist and partner extraordinaire, and Dr. Wayne Hunt, who collaborated with me on a paraphilia project, and both of whom have continued to tolerate working with me all these years.

Dr. Jeffery Hsu, Dr. Adam Kaplin, Ms. Olivia Radcliffe, Mr. Jack Bonner, and Ms. Suzanne Cannon joined our group several years ago, and without their help we would have failed in our efforts. We were also able to attract a series of wonderful colleagues, including Dr. Adam Rosenblatt, Dr. Joseph Schwartz, Dr. Jean Driscoll, Dr. Susan Patania, Mr. Joe Hickey, and Ms. Carolyn Gorman. Several others have worked with us over the years for extended periods of time, including Dr. Anne Hanson, Dr. Chiadi Onyike, Dr. Duncan Cameron, Mr. Nicholas Schweizer, Dr. Katherine Neel, Dr. Fred Schaerf, Ms. Nicole Rohrer, Ms. Heidi Block, Ms. Kelly Pac, Dr. Todd Cox, Dr. Richard Carpenter, and Mr. Tom Eversole. Last, Dr. Andy Angelino returned from Denver to join the faculty at Johns Hopkins and help me (GT) with my work. I am forever in his debt, for without him I would never have completed this book.

Dr. Adam Kaplin, not long after he joined our group, and after a particularly "interesting" clinic, reminded me of the Talmudic phrase, "He who saves one life, it is as if he saves the whole world." This is also quoted in the main hallway at Johns Hopkins Hospital. It lacks glamour, but these are the words my partners have lived by these 14 years. The key is that they have not quit. These are the trenches, and instead of pursuing well-funded Ivory Tower projects that yield fame and fortune, these clinicians have waded into the mud of psychiatric illness and dragged patients out one at a time. It is hard work, but it is good work.

We wish to thank and acknowledge the contributions to this work of our friends and colleagues. We thank Dr. Andrew Tompkins for a critical reading and editing of the manuscript. Dr. Joyce King and Dr. Jennifer Riedinger read this manuscript and made extensive helpful comments; moreover, they remained married to us and did not kick us out of our homes during the writing of this book. Our mentors, Dr. Paul McHugh, the most visionary and clear-thinking psychiatrist of our time, and Dr. John Bartlett, the greatest AIDS doctor who will ever live, have been a support, inspiration, and endless source of good sense and direction. Both have been patient teachers and giant shoulders to stand on or cry on, depending on the day.

We also wish to thank our colleagues in the world of HIV care who have supported our work and helped us. Although such a list will always be incomplete and we apologize to anyone we have left out, we wish to thank Karla Alwood, Jean Anderson, Patricia Barditch-Crovo, William Bishai, Robert Bollinger, Joseph Brady, Heather Campbell, Clara Chaisson, Lelia Chaisson, Richard Chaisson, Laura Cheever, Joe Cofrancesco, Lawrence Deyton, Emily Erbelding, Joe Eron, Ian Everall, Judith Feinberg, Charles Flexner, Ian Frank, Joel Gallant, John Gerwig, Rebecca Godfrey, Jane Houck, Doug Jabs, Jean Keller, William Kelly, Newton Kendig, Jeanne Keruly, Debra Kosco, George Larson, Jo Marie Leslie, Arlette Lindsay, Greg Lucas, Janine Maenza, Justin McArthur, Robin McKenzie, John Mann, Anna Mullins, Ciro Martins, Richard Moore, Joe O'Neill, Milan Nermut, Michael Paradise, John Phair, Peggy Piazza, Tom Quinn, Charles Raines, Anne Rampalo, Stuart Ray, William Ruby, Susan Rucker, Michael Saag, Cynthia Sears, Robert Siliciano, Tim Sterling, Aruna Subramanian, Mark Sulkowski, Dave Thomas, Charles Van der Horst, Lisa Wolf, Wesla Zeller, and Jon Zenilman. I again apologize to those whose names were omitted from this list but who have helped us in this work, my level of disorganization will surely have made me miss many of you. The work in this book could not have been accomplished without your support.

Lastly, we are living proof that behind every man who looks successful there is a woman keeping him that way. While we pledge our undying love and gratitude to our wives, Ms. Emmera Wheeler has proven herself to be the definition of perfection as a secretary. She keeps us looking better than we ought to, tirelessly fussing over and supporting us. We are incredibly fortunate to have her.

—Glenn Treisman

Quotes from the Clinic

Thank you for saving my life, Dr. Treisman. Can I have a dollar?

Why did you miss your last appointment here at the clinic?
It was snowing.
Would you have gone out to "cop" if you were using?
Of course.
Well, you have to be willing to go out in worse weather to get sober than you would to "cop," because it is harder to get sober than to stay an addict.

I have been very nervous lately because I have been buying cocaine from a guy who shot me.
Why do you buy cocaine from a guy who shot you?
Because he has cocaine.
I really like prime rib, but if the maitre d' at the Prime Rib restaurant shot me, I wouldn't go there any more.
With a [sic] attitude like that, you could miss out on some really good meat.

I know what helps me. Valium helps me.
You have been using Valium for years and you live in a refrigerator box. I don't think the Valium is helping you.
OK, how about Xanax?

When I shoot coke into my pulse vein (the carotid artery), I get a bad headache on one side of my head. What have you got for headaches?

I hate this clinic and I hate this disease. First of all, there is no food here.

I would love to help you, Dr. Treisman, but what you are asking is just impossible with my current schedule.

Drug treatment is a good concept, but it doesn't work for me.

I don't need to see a shrink. I just need new virus medicine.
But the doctors who see you say you are not taking the medicine right and that you have a resistant virus that is very hard to treat.
I'll take it right this time.
Aren't you the guy who got sick in the waiting room last week because you were in withdrawal from heroin?
Yes.

You're not even compliant with heroin, and you're addicted to it. How do you think you can remember to take antiviral medications? You need to do some work first.

I have heard about you, Dr. Treisman. I think we will get along better if you know that I am not going to do anything you say.

Tylox, Pecocet, Vicodan, Oxycontin, and them patches — I tried them all and ain't none of them done nothing for my pain. Which one you gonna give me?

What drug do you take so you can work here?

Dr. Treisman, are you still working here? How come you ain't burned out yet?

That medicine you give me give me side effects.
What side effects?
A dry mouth.
Cocaine gave you a stroke, and you still take that.
Yeah, but that makes me feel good.
My medicine made you feel good after you took it for a while.
Yeah, but it takes too long.

Dr. Treisman, did you ever shoot cocaine?
No, because I could end up addicted.
But it feels so good.
I could get HIV.
Yeah, but it feels so good.
I could end up with an abscess like the one that you have on your leg.
Yeah, I can see why we can't communicate.

[From a one-armed patient:] I woulda lost my other arm, too, but once you lost your arm, it's really hard to shoot up in your one arm, so I got to use other places. I'm worried I will lose my leg.

I need to get out of this hospital today so I can get my check cashed and use my money before my mother gets it and uses it for my rent and bills.

I don't want to get a payee. Then I won't have any of my money.
Where is your money now?
I spent it all on drugs.

My way might be crazy, but it's how I've always done it.

You're smart. Add up all the money you have spent on drugs in the last 10 years. How much do you use in a day?

Forty dollars.

And multiply that by 365 days a year.

About fourteen thousand. [In about three seconds, he did the math.]

And multiply that by 10 years.

About a hundred and forty thousand.

Do you think that's about right?

No, spent more than that, because of coke and other stuff.

Where do you think the money went?

I don't know.

Anyone in your neighborhood been killed in a drive-by shooting?

Yeah.

Any children?

Yeah.

Did you ever think you might have paid for the bullet?

I never thought of it.

And you paid for the lawyer so the guy could get out of jail and do it again.

Yeah, and his flashy car and them guns. Yeah, I get what you're saying. Yeah, makes me sick. All that bread, I could've bought a McDonald's. That's a lot of bread to spend on destroying your own people. All right, sign me up for whatever. Yeah, you got me. I never thought of that kid thing. Yeah, that's so heavy. Yeah, I won't do it no more. We lost a kid right on my block. Okay. All right, now you got me to crying. Fine. I'll go to group, but I don't think it's fair how you did that, but yeah, I'll go, 'cause you right. I don't think you should do people the way you did me, but you right. Cold, but you right. You cold, Dr. T, cold. Where was you 10 years ago to tell us that shit?

I need Tylox.

No, you like Tylox; you need air. If you don't get air, you die. If you don't get Tylox, you are uncomfortable. Do you see the difference between need and want?

I can't stop using drugs.

No, you won't stop using drugs. If I had a gun pointed at you, and there were drugs on the table, and I told you I would shoot you if you used the drugs, would you use the drugs?

I don't know.

What if I shot off a toe just to let you know I was serious?

Yeah, then I could keep from using. But to tell the truth, you probably would have to shoot a toe off to make me know you were serious.

I can't go to group.
Can't *means* won't. *If I give you 50 dollars, will you go to group?*
Yes.
How much did you spend on drugs and alcohol this week?
About 200.
*If you go to group and stay sober, you will have 200 dollars you won't have if you
    don't go to group, and I will give you your medicines, too.*

My girlfriend left me, so I want to kill her.
Why did she leave you?
She didn't want to go down in the road anymore.
*She didn't want to work as a prostitute to pay for your drug habit anymore, so she
    left you?*
Yeah.
Do you hear how ridiculous that sounds?
Yeah, when you say it, it sounds ridiculous, but that's how I feel.

Dr. Treisman, can I borrow 10 dollars?
No, you know I never give money to patients.
Then can I have some crackers and juice?
If there is any in the kitchen, I will get some for you.
Then can I have five dollars?
No.
All right, see about the crackers and juice.

*[To a patient with no limbs from congenital malformation:] You are addicted to
    IV heroin?*
Yes.
How do you manage to shoot up?
I just ask somebody to shoot the drugs for me.
You need to surround yourself with people who say, "No."

*[After a patient had a tantrum in the clinic and lit himself on fire in the bathroom,
    he was discharged from the clinic. He wanted to know why he was being dis-
    charged.]*
*You are a fire hazard. There is oxygen in this clinic, and you endangered the lives
    of everyone here. I can't help you if you are willing to hurt yourself and every-
    one around you just to express your feelings.*

I only use heroin for medical reasons. For me, it's just a medicine, like penicillin.

*When you tell me I am a drug addict, that makes me feel bad. You're a psychiatrist.
    You're supposed to make people feel better.*
*No, I am a doctor. I am supposed to help people get better. It is the unrelenting
    search for feeling good that made you an addict in the first place.*

When you came into the hospital, how far could you walk?
About across my bedroom.
And were you on more pain medicines then or now?
I'm off almost all my pain medicines now.
And can you walk farther or less far?
Oh, I can walk a long way now.
And is your pain worse now or when you came in?
My pain is better now.
See — do more, feel better. Do more, feel better. Take less medicine, feel better. Do more, feel better. Now you say it.

Chapter One
Why AIDS Psychiatry?

The essential thesis of this book is that human immunodeficiency virus (HIV) infection has become a psychiatric epidemic. HIV both causes and exacerbates psychiatric disorders, and the presence of a psychiatric disorder leads to an increased risk of infection with HIV and worsens someone's prognosis once he or she is infected.

The goal of this text is to describe the relationship between psychiatric disorders and the HIV epidemic, and to demonstrate how the effective recognition and treatment of mental disorders can improve the care of HIV-infected persons. The psychiatric disorders include those caused by HIV as well as preexisting disorders that complicate the treatment and prevention of HIV. Many think that the work of psychiatry in an HIV clinic centers on grief counseling, reassurance, and emotional support for persons infected with HIV. However, patients must be counseled before testing, be educated about risks, overcome the traumatic effect of diagnosis, conquer barriers in intimate and family relationships, adapt to living with HIV, and develop strategies for taking on a huge burden of medications and treatments. They need help with death and dying but even more help with living. Many health care providers already excel at these elements of care, and many authors have discussed these issues in relation to HIV and other disorders, as they are not unique to this epidemic. Although we review this material in the latter part of the book, we also emphasize the elements of the epidemic that are unique to the interaction between HIV infection and psychiatric disorders.

Initially, HIV was a disorder that affected persons who did not know that their behavior placed them at risk for a potentially fatal disease. The epidemic began at a time of increased cultural tolerance and decreased sexual restraint, and therefore intravenous drug use and sexual contact with multiple partners spread the epidemic rapidly in communities where these behaviors were prevalent. These patients had psychiatric disorders at higher than expected rates, which was believed to be because of HIV's effect on both the brain and the life of the person. Later in the epidemic, after the risk factors were elucidated, widespread public education was directed at prevention. At this time a new principle began to operate: psychiatric disorders were recognized as major impediments to some individuals' ability to modify their behavior to prevent infection. Moreover, as effective treatments for HIV became available and patient care shifted from terminal to earlier stages of the disease, psychiatric disorders were recognized as severely complicating treatment. These principles operate in tandem to fuel the epidemic spread of HIV now.

Fig. 1.1 demonstrates that the HIV virus, as it causes damage to the brain and creates turmoil in the lives of infected persons, causes or exacerbates psychiatric disorders. Further, psychiatric disorders, as they disorganize behavior, decrease a person's ability to effectively change behavior and thus increase the risk of infection and morbidity.

Currently, many persons who contract HIV in North America, western Europe, and, to a lesser extent, many other areas of the world can be described as "vulnerable." This vulnerability derives from some disorder of a psychiatric nature. This may be as fundamental as an illness, such as major depression or a bipolar disorder, or as obvious as the result of geographical, financial, social, or some other disenfranchisement from the rest of the population. These vulnerable people continue to practice high-risk behaviors at high rates despite public

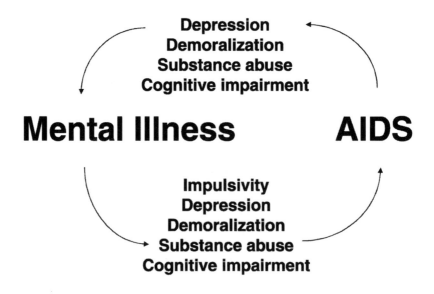

Fig. 1.1. A self-perpetuating cycle of increasing morbidity: mental illness and AIDS

education about the risks of what they are doing—and often despite having seen someone they know afflicted by or even die of acquired immunodeficiency syndrome (AIDS).

Although substantial data support this point, the data from our group at Johns Hopkins provide a specific example. In a survey of patients at their first appointment for HIV care, we found the primary diagnoses shown in Table 1.1. Although some authors initially reported lower prevalences than these, over time the number of persons with psychiatric disorders in HIV clinics has continued to rise. Each disorder in Table 1.1 is an example of mental illness as shown in Fig. 1.1, thus driving the cycle of the epidemic.

This is not to say that everyone infected or becoming infected is psychiatrically ill. Many patients live in an area of high prevalence of HIV infection and, in the course of modest risk, become infected. Condom use and safer sex practices, as well as needle exchange and bleach needle cleaning programs, have had a large influence, effectively changing behaviors for many people. However, sexual activity and needle use, even with these precautions, can be associated with "slips" and mechanical failures. Research on infection as the result of such a failure is extremely difficult to perform. Given the available data, however, it is clear that the majority of persons who become infected in the United States engage in high rates of risky behaviors that are associated with the vulnerabilities seen in psychiatric disorders.

In addition to increasing the risk of infection, psychiatric disorders decrease patients' ability to gain access to medical care. First, psychiatric disorders directly disorganize patients and make them feel hopeless, diminishing their effectiveness and desire to seek medical attention. Second, the medical treatment of persons with psychiatric problems is more complex and time consuming. Primary care doctors are not adequately trained to diagnose and treat mental illness, and tertiary care subspecialists, in infectious diseases, for example, have even less

Table 1.1. Primary diagnoses of patients at first appointment for HIV care (N = 250)

Primary Diagnosis	%
Any Axis I psychiatric disturbance (other than substance use disorder)	54
Major Depression	20
Adjustment Disorder (all types)	18
Cognitive Impairment	18
Substance Use Disorder	74
Personality Disorder (all types)	26

training in this regard. Health care providers are often baffled and overwhelmed by mentally ill persons, and do not know how to integrate medical and mental health care. Third, many mentally ill persons are economically disadvantaged. They often are "carved out" by managed care organizations, so their care is fragmented. They are then sent to different clinics and even different institutions to receive care.

Last, psychiatric disorders have a negative effect on a person's adherence to medical care. This in turn often negatively affects both health care providers' subjective experience of caring for very vulnerable patients and the statistical outcomes of treatment. To prevent viral resistance, and therefore treatment failure, patients must consistently take at least 90 percent of their prescribed antiretroviral medications.[1,2] These medications not only improve patient's health but also decrease the amount of virus in the blood, making patients less infectious. Depression and substance abuse interfere with patients' adherence to treatment regimens,[3] and other psychiatric disorders likely interfere in a less direct way. The best outcomes that have been demonstrated in trials of HIV antiviral treatment give rates of sustained, undetectable viral load in 75 to 85 percent of subjects, but these trials used research-subject populations where psychiatric disorders have been minimized by screening or by the rigors of study enrollment. However, in clinical settings with patients with no exclusions, including persons with psychiatric disorders as described, the rate of sustained viral suppression has been shown to be in the 25–40 percent range.[4]

The effective recognition and treatment of psychiatric disorders in an HIV clinic can overcome these problems. To achieve this, psychiatric services in HIV clinics are directed at three primary goals:

- Improved quality of life for persons with HIV. The treatment of psychiatric disorders results in reduced psychiatric symptoms and improved function. Patients can work, engage in relationships, enjoy activities, and live more independently. They feel better, and they live better.

- Increased ability to tolerate and engage in medical treatment. The treatment of psychiatric disorders leads to better adherence to medical regimens and scheduled medical appointments. Alleviating psychiatric symptoms leads to a better foundation for medical treatment because of improved function. Patients with resources obtain better treatment, and patients in relationships have the necessary support to help them with difficult treatment. They also have more reasons to live longer and to work at caring for themselves.

- Decreased risk for transmitting HIV. Patients responding to psychiatric treatment are better organized and able to engage in preventive measures. Patients who are no longer depressed take better care of themselves and those who are no longer addicted to drugs have better control over their relationships and sexual lives.

The results of these interventions benefit the patients, the medical team, and society as a whole. The patients have improved outcomes, and the medical team members develop a sense of satisfaction and therapeutic optimism for the care of patients. Decreased propagation of the epidemic improves the general human condition.

The most common psychiatric disorders seen in an HIV clinic are shown in Table 1.1. Major depression, AIDS dementia, schizophrenia, and bipolar disorder are discussed in the first section of this book. The second section covers problems of temperament and personality. Substance use disorders are discussed in the third section, along with disorders of sexuality and paraphilia. Demoralization (called Adjustment Disorder in the *Diagnostic and Statistical Manual of Mental Disorders* [DSM])[5] and other extreme reactions to life circumstances are discussed in the fourth section. The final section of the book addresses the issues of health care provider burnout, therapeutic nihilism, and integration of care.

Funding Mental Health Care for HIV Patients

At present, the United States is facing potentially the worst epidemic in human history, and yet health care is rationed. A huge part of the U.S. health care budget is going to administration. Insurance companies and the government pay legions of people to review health care, to prevent payments for health care, to search for Medicare fraud, and to monitor health care costs. This means that doctors, hospitals, and clinics must also pay legions of people to fight to get paid, to argue with insurers, and to defend doctors' decisions. In the midst of this contentious environment, persons who are mentally ill, disenfranchised, poor, geographically and socially isolated, substance abusing, cognitively impaired, and HIV infected have little or no chance. They have no voice, do not vote, are disorganized and desperate, and have few champions.

There is an increasing sense that some patients can be discarded, are too hard or expensive to save, or consume too many resources. Critics of the medical care system emphasize that 14 percent of the gross national product is spent on health care. They fail to mention that, although the efforts to control the costs of medical care have not resulted in decreased costs, they have resulted in a dramatic decrease in the delivery of medical care. Resources are being redirected from medical care to the administrative costs of regulating care.

The media and the insurers have popularized the view that callous doctors milking millions from the medical system are extending thousands of lives in a meaningless way. The fictional idea that hospitals have hundreds of comatose patients on ventilators is an example of this exaggeration. Most persons who are mortally ill die rapidly, despite medical intervention. In a study of intensive care in England, an instrument for predicting death—the APACHE II scale—was used to predict which patients in intensive care units would die. All patients in the study received full care despite the prediction that they would die. Of the patients predicted to die, almost all died within 2 days, but 5 percent survived and went on to have a good quality of life.[6] A conclusion this study reached was that intensive care costs could be saved, but at the cost of one life in twenty.

Several important points support our efforts to treat and save patients with difficult-to-treat disorders and uncertain outcomes. The first is the progress made in extending the frontiers of medicine. Breast cancer survival is no longer science fiction, but a reality of modern health care. Patients receive what are essentially fatal doses of chemotherapy and then are rescued medically with bone marrow transplants and other interventions. Advances in intensive care medicine, the result of caring for "futile" outcome patients, have resulted in the technology to make these treatments possible. Even a few years ago, these patients would have died from treatments that are routine today.

The AIDS epidemic is a great example of this as well. The aggressive treatment of opportunistic infections has resulted in research that developed new techniques, such as aerosolized pentamidine. Five new classes of antiviral drugs with several drugs in three classes have been developed as well. The success of antiretroviral medications for HIV has created a new enthusiasm for viral treatment. Millions of dollars and thousands of lives can now be saved because of the development of effective treatment for hepatitis C and the decreased reliance on liver transplants. Several of the drugs developed for HIV are currently in trials for the treatment of other conditions.

The second reason to treat patients with an uncertain outcome is that ultimately it is cheaper than the alternative. Patients who receive effective care for HIV are better able to care for themselves, function at work and in social settings, and require fewer medical services. Additionally, the decreased level of virus in the blood of a successfully treated person decreases the probability of infecting others, with the attendant cost of treating new infections if the person continues to engage in unsafe behaviors.

The addition of comprehensive mental health care to an AIDS clinic may well be the most cost-effective effort available. Psychiatric services can be added to most clinic settings for as little as a few hundred dollars per month, saving thousands of dollars on each patient who becomes more adherent to antiviral therapy. Patients who respond to treatment for mental illness become far easier to treat and have a far better quality of life. Treatment is also more efficient when patients come to their appointments on time, and care is less disjointed when fewer disruptive emergency visits occur and when misuse of the hospital emergency department for emotional crises is less frequent. Members of the medical care team are consequently buoyed by the improved patients, resulting in less cost to medical centers for the treatment, and possibly replacement, of burned-out health care providers. Most important, the treatment of mental illness decreases high-risk behaviors, which acts synergistically with decreases in the viral load within the community to oppose the epidemic.

The third reason to treat patients with an uncertain outcome is that it is the right thing to do. Ultimately, the medical profession is altruistic and directed at providing care for those who are vulnerable, ill, and suffering. It is not a matter of proving that health care is economically advantageous, despite the widespread demand that it must be, as propagated by administrators of the U.S. health care dollar. The idea that care for a patient must be "medically necessary" to warrant reimbursement (that is, the patient will die without it) is a new and altered standard in health care. It must be supplanted by the older idea of "medically beneficial," which suggests we will do what helps people to live full and recovered lives whenever possible. Advances in medical science result in qualitative societal improvements that are impossible to quantify accurately, just as stock analysts often cite "good economic feelings" for increases in the market but are unable to predict a percentage rise from the morning mood of a certain company's CEO.

Currently, health service provisions for most psychiatrically ill persons are deplorable. In HIV clinics, collaborative and subspecialty mental health treatment is the exception rather than the rule. Drug-addicted, psychiatrically ill persons often receive the least medical care and poor psychiatric care. This is despite the substantial evidence reviewed throughout this book that this group is currently a major vector of HIV infection in the United States and that effective treatment significantly influences the outcome of these patients.

This book's purpose is to emphasize that care for these complicated but treatable patients must be improved. This effort is worthwhile, is productive, and can be accomplished by clinicians. Using the models and point-by-point guidance found in this text, clinicians can understand and effectively treat persons with complicated psychiatric diagnoses, improving their outcomes. Further, with effective skills in caring for these severely ill persons, health care providers will reap great rewards, are more likely to find their work satisfying and enjoyable, and are less likely to burn out. Finally, our efforts to stop HIV will be increasingly fruitful when the very psychiatric disorders that drive behaviors that perpetuate the epidemic are recognized and treated in HIV clinics.

AIDS 101 for Mental Health Professionals

This section outlines the history of HIV and AIDS treatment and the changes that have occurred in the epidemic, particularly those elements that are relevant to mental health issues. The epidemic that we now face has infected 33 million people worldwide. In the United States, there are approximately 1 million infected persons. The virus infects immune cells in the body, particularly macrophages and T-helper (CD4) lymphocytes, rapidly multiplying and killing infected cells. The virus was identified in the mid-1980s, but probably originated as an infection in human beings as early as the 1950s and began to spread in an epidemic way in the 1970s.[7] Since the beginning of the epidemic, several important changes have greatly affected the treatment of infected persons. These changes can be seen in the following historical context.

The Era of Palliation

The first era of AIDS care began with the initial case descriptions and ended with the ability to identify HIV-infected persons before the development of AIDS. During this time, treatment was directed at patient comfort and the prevention and treatment of opportunistic infections. Research was focused on finding an etiology and source of the illness.

The first cases of AIDS were reported in the early 1980s. Physicians were puzzled by the presence of rare infections and conditions in seemingly healthy young homosexual men. The infections were remarkable in that they had previously been described only in severely immunocompromised persons. Pneumonia from *Pneumocystis carinii*, a common organism that rarely causes infection, and invasive Kaposi sarcoma, an unusual cancer that was ordinarily localized and relatively circumscribed, were noticed early. Several cases were published and the search for the relationship between cases was sought. Even early on, an infectious etiology was suspected.

By the mid-1980s, AIDS was recognized as an epidemic infection causing an acquired immune deficiency and was characterized as being spread by intimate contact. Risk groups included the so-called 4-H club: *homosexual* men, people from *Haiti*, intravenous drug users (*heroin*), frequent transfusion recipients (*hemophilia*), and *health* care workers (yes, there were five). The general public feared infection from casual contact, but no evidence was found to support this. Researchers diligently pursued a viral etiologic agent, and the candidate virus, initially called human T-lymphocyte virus (HTLV) and later renamed human immunodeficiency virus (HIV), was finally characterized.

In the scientific community, however, a debate arose as to the cause of AIDS, and even years after the virus was identified, debate continued as to whether HIV was the true etiologic agent for AIDS. Over time, increasing numbers of patients presented with catastrophic opportunistic infections. The prognosis was grim, and previously healthy young patients rapidly wasted away. Even when the initial opportunistic infection responded to treatment, most patients died within months of another infection or a recurrence. Therefore, clinicians directed their efforts at palliative care.

At this time, much of the focus of care was on patients in terminal stages. Limited therapeutic options were available, and professionals often felt overwhelmed by the needs and losses of their patients. Many professionals burned out, as described by Abraham Verghese in his book *My Own Country*,[8] because of the apparent futility of seeing so many deaths with so little to offer patients. The critical development during this phase of the epidemic was the widespread implementation of hospice and comfort care. Weary providers often created support groups and other strategies for coping with the losses associated with AIDS.

The Era of Therapeutic Monitoring

The first major changes in the epidemic came with widespread understanding and public education about the behaviors that led to a high risk of infection. Changes also occurred as a result of the development of the ability to detect infection before immunosuppression. Serologic testing that could reveal the presence of infection in asymptomatic persons was developed in the mid-1980s and could warn patients of the risk of infecting others. The stages of disease were also defined: acute infection, asymptomatic HIV infection, symptomatic HIV infection, and AIDS. AIDS still had a grim prognosis, but advances in the treatment of opportunistic infection led to the testing of prophylactic treatments for immunosuppressed patients. This not only extended patients' lives but also gave purpose to the clinical investigation of patients and their outcomes. The focus of treatment shifted from comfort care to preventing both opportunistic infections and the epidemic spread of HIV infections.

Commensurate with this was the discovery that HIV selectively depleted T-helper lymphocyte (CD4) cells and that the vulnerability to opportunistic infections correlated with CD4 counts. Equipped with this new tool, physicians learned when to begin prophylactic treatments. Fig. 1.2 shows the average course of an HIV infection. Although at first glance it was a grim map of impending death, it gave patients and physicians a way to plan treatment, structure goals for treatment, and measure the results of interventions.

This era was accompanied by a change in the patient population. Earlier in the epidemic, people did not know that certain behaviors subjected them to a potentially fatal illness. Now, with widespread publicity about HIV risk behaviors, people could decrease their risk by altering their behavior. The gay men in large cities began to organize and educate their communities. Efforts toward the use of clean needles and condoms were directed at high-risk persons. People at risk who were able to modify their behavior slowly began to do just that.

This meant a change in the character of many HIV clinics. Previously, the patient population was largely gay white men. Because the gay community was

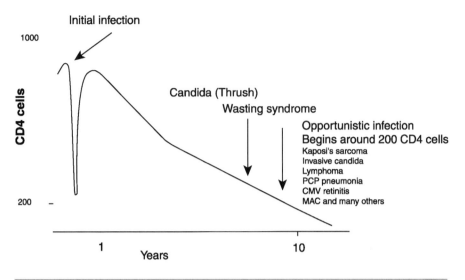

Fig. 1.2. The average course of HIV infection

successful in its educational efforts to decrease risky behavior, as the initial cohort of these patients died and fewer gay men presented with new cases of HIV infection, intravenous drug-using patients became the majority of new patients. Additionally, sexually acquired HIV spread more widely among heterosexual populations. Specifically, subgroups such as those involved in prostitution, sexual partners of injecting drug users, and people with large numbers of sexual partners began to be a significant vector of infection. Public health initiatives consequently broadened the scope of the efforts at prevention.

One of the important changes associated with this era was the increase in the length of time patients were followed in the clinics. This was due in part to increased survival time for persons with AIDS. Persons with advanced disease benefited from prophylactic treatment and could expect to survive an increasing number of opportunistic infections. The question of when to stop became a hotly debated and important topic. Further, clinics followed patients for months to years because of the earlier detection of infection. Persons with CD4 counts of greater than 200 and without active illness could receive monitoring, counseling, and rehabilitative treatment for addictions and high-risk behaviors. The discovery of coinfection with other sexually transmitted diseases made the prevention of risk behavior personally relevant to infected persons and thus something more than altruism and community sovereignty.

Often, persons presenting at early stages of the disease received confusing messages from health care providers. The therapeutic nihilism of earlier experiences with persons with AIDS, along with an inability to predict the rapid advance of antiviral therapy, made many health care providers emphasize the apparent futility of treatment. In retrospect, it is easy to see how important therapeutic optimism was at that critical time, but it is also understandable that practitioners found it difficult to be optimistic. In the worst scenarios, clinicians gave patients comfort measures too soon, persuaded by the climate of pessimism and the patients' demands. In some clinics, huge quantities of addictive substances were prescribed for sedation, and some patients even feigned HIV infection to get into clinics where access to controlled substances was readily available.

Toward the end of this era, from the late 1980s into the early 1990s, the role of psychiatric disorders in the HIV epidemic was recognized. Several studies described the prevalence of disorders other than emotional reactions to the illness, including mood disorders, personality disorders, and addictions.[9] Further, brain injuries and other consequences of HIV were hypothesized to play a role in the etiology of some psychiatric disorders. Supportive care and counseling had long been a part of most clinics, but psychopharmacologic and psychotherapeutic interventions were required for these complicated patients. A few leaders in HIV psychiatry emerged who described how mood disorders, dementia, substance abuse, and personality disorders could lead to risky behaviors. People who were able to change their lives in response to public education on HIV risks did so, whereas other people became infected because of some barrier to behavioral change. HIV had become a disorder of a subpopulation vulnerable to high-risk behavior.

The Era of Viral Suppression

The era of viral suppression occurred in two stages. The first stage was the parallel development of new antiretroviral drugs and new insights into the virology and pathology of HIV. The second stage was the rational discovery that multidrug regimens, or combined therapies, resulted in robust and vigorous viral suppression that could be sustained for indefinite periods of treatment.

In the late 1980s and early 1990s, several new drugs made their way from the laboratory to the clinical care of persons with HIV. Azidothymidine (AZT), now called Zidovudine, is a nucleoside analog and inhibits the enzyme reverse transcriptase (see Figs. 1.3, 1.4). The class is now known as nucleoside analog reverse transcriptase inhibitors (NRTIs, or "nukes").

This drug was a breakthrough in several ways. First, as an antiviral drug, it was strong evidence against the widely held belief that only vaccines and immunotherapies could fight viruses and that drugs like Amantadine and Acyclovir were flukes. Second, it was a great example of rational drug design. The

The Psychiatry of AIDS

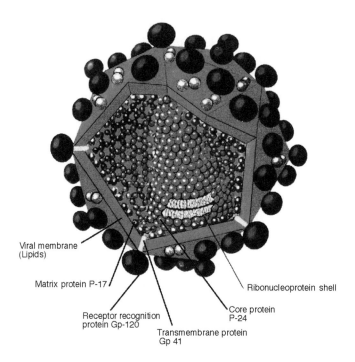

Viral membrane
(Lipids)

Matrix protein P-17

Receptor recognition
protein Gp-120

Transmembrane protein
Gp 41

Core protein
P-24

Ribonucleoprotein shell

Fig. 1.3. The HIV viral particle

HIV virus is called a retrovirus, as its genetic material is carried in ribonucleic acid (RNA) form instead of a deoxyribonucleic acid (DNA) form. To infect cells, the viral RNA must be made into DNA first. This is a process that does not normally occur in human cells.

DNA and RNA are typically both made from a cell's existing DNA template, and no enzyme in normal cells can make the reverse process occur to make DNA from RNA. The RNA viruses must carry their own enzymes to circumvent this problem, and in the case of many RNA viruses, that enzyme is called reverse transcriptase (some RNA viruses use other ways to replicate their RNA). Drugs that inhibit reverse transcriptase inhibit HIV viral replication.

Although AZT can affect other enzymes, its effect at reverse transcriptase would essentially affect only viral replication, not normal cell function. Despite the later finding that the virus rapidly mutated to become resistant to AZT (within about six months), AZT gave patients about 18 months of additional life. A series of drugs, d4T (Stavudine), ddI (Didanosine), ddC (Zalcitabine), and 3TC (Lamivudine), that all work by the same mechanism were promptly developed.

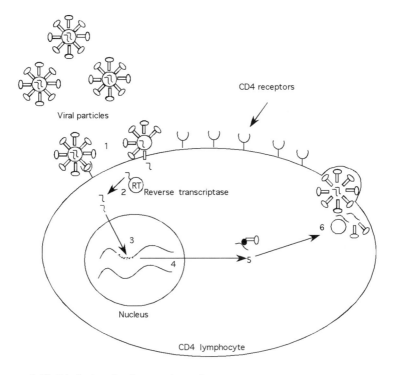

1 Viral binding to cell surface receptors and
  internalization of viral content
  (SITE OF ACTION OF FUSION INHIBITORS)
2 Reverse transcriptase makes viral DNA
  (SITE OF ACTION OF NNRTIs and NRTIs)
3 Viral integration into host genome
4 Transcription of DNA to RNA
5 Translation of viral RNA to protein components
6 Protein processing, cleavage, viral assembly, and budding
  (SITE OF ACTION OF PROTEASE INHIBITORS)

Fig. 1.4. The figure shows the life cycle of the HIV virus as it infects and destroys a susceptible cell. Viral particles bind to CD4 receptors found on the surface of T lymphocytes (and macrophages) and are internalized, and the viral RNA and enzymes are released into the cell. The viral enzyme reverse transcriptase makes DNA transcripts of the RNA strand, which are then carried to the nucleus where they are further transcribed back to RNA by the cell's own machinery. The RNA is then used to make the viral proteins necessary for particles, and the finished proteins are assembled into viral particles by the cell. Finally a protease cleaves them to activate them into infectious viral particles.

Source: Treisman and Angelino (with thanks to Milan Nermut for his helpful comments)

The development of antiviral drugs was greatly encouraging. Although many cited the development of viral resistance and felt AZT was not a real gain, others saw better treatments on the horizon. Hope blossomed both in patients, who now had a real medication to fight the virus, and in health care providers, who now had a treatment aimed at the virus, not merely at its aftermath. A renewed enthusiasm ensued about diagnostic testing, which up to this point had mostly served the purpose of epidemic control. Finding infected persons was seen to have more direct benefit, as treatment was available to slow the progression of disease.

Originally, HIV was thought to be a "slow" virus with an indolent course (it is part of a family called lentivirus, meaning slow virus). The quick development of resistance to AZT was difficult to explain. Two important new discoveries aided in reconciling this paradox. The first was the ability to quantitatively measure the viral particles in blood, described as viral load.[10] This led to the realization that the actual amounts of virus present were extremely variable and often huge. The average infection produces 10 billion viral particles each day. The amount of the virus in blood was found to directly predict how fast the CD4 count would diminish and how quickly HIV would progress. The second discovery was related: the body makes vast numbers of CD4 cells every day.[11]

This explained the resistance phenomenon. Ten billion viral particles turn over every day in an infected person, and point mutation variants of the virus are constantly being made. HIV is not a slow, indolent killer that the body cannot fight. Instead, a huge war between the immune system and the virus occurs every minute a person is infected. The immune system loses to this malignant virus in a war of gradual attrition.

The treatment of HIV in this era (before 1995) was the sequential use of anti-retroviral agents as resistance developed to each subsequent drug. Two new classes of drugs were on the horizon: the protease inhibitors (PIs) and the non-nucleoside reverse transcriptase inhibitors (NNRTIs, or "non-nukes"). These new drugs were also clearly vulnerable to the hasty development of viral resist-ance. Before trials of combined agents, most clinicians assumed that therapy would involve a race to develop new treatments just as old treatments gave out.

All of this was dramatically changed by the findings announced at the Inter-national AIDS Conference at Vancouver in 1995. Several trials reported that year showed that the administration of three drug combination regimens, con-sisting of two nucleoside reverse transcriptase analogs and a protease inhibitor, resulted in a dramatic reduction in the viral load. In fact, the viral reduction was so profound that in some patients no viral particles were detectable. This was accompanied in many patients by an increase in the CD4 count. The duration of the response was predicted by how completely the virus was suppressed.

This made sense, given what was now known about HIV. As long as signifi-cant viral replication was occurring, significant numbers of mutations leading to drug resistance would occur. But if viral replication was suppressed almost com-pletely, the virus could not "escape" therapy because it could not produce sufficient mutations to develop resistance. The end result was a marked increase in patient survival, as demonstrated in several studies.[12-14]

The stage was set for the current dilemma faced by HIV health care providers. As stated earlier, the current regimens of antiviral therapy (referred to as highly active antiretroviral therapy, or HAART) can achieve vigorous suppression in 75–85 percent of drug-naive research subjects, but in far fewer real-world patients in clinical settings. This is partly a matter of drug exposure, pharmacodynamics, and viral resistance, but it is mostly a matter of getting patients to take their medications accurately and consistently. An effective and sustained viral suppression requires that at least 90 percent of the medication be taken as directed. With these premises, the problem that is easily derived states, "How does one get a real-life patient to be as adherent to the medication regimen as a research subject and thus achieve the high rate of success?"

The State of the Art

HIV treatment now consists of a complicated set of variables that may make it a subspecialty on its own. Although treatments are changing so quickly that it may be difficult to keep up, the principles that follow will likely continue to provide a general outline for therapy. There are four stages of HIV infection.

Exposure

At this point, a certain number of viral particles are introduced to a vulnerable tissue. Direct blood contact, such as transfusion or the injection of contaminated blood, has a very high likelihood of producing an infection. Sexual exposure in a single event has a relatively lower risk, unless there is trauma or a coexisting infection. Given population data, mixed opinion exists as to whether or not to give post-exposure prophylaxis after a sexual encounter if the HIV status of the partner is unknown. The best data come from newborns, who have dramatically lower rates of HIV infection if they receive prophylaxis or if their mothers are treated with AZT alone before delivery.[15] Health care workers tracked after needle stick exposure show lower rates of infection if given post-exposure treatment.[16] Because little evidence suggests that short-term treatment causes severe or long-lasting toxicity in most patients, aggressive treatments may be encouraged. The CDC guidelines recommend treatment in high-risk exposures but are less supportive of prophylaxis in low-risk exposures.

Acute Viral Infection

Acute HIV infection is accompanied by a dramatic fall in CD4 counts, a flu-like illness with occasional encephalitis-like features, very rare cases of Guillain-Barré syndrome, and the development of HIV-directed antibodies (seroconversion). When patients present at this stage, which is somewhat unusual, treatment is mostly supportive, although some clinicians advocate for aggressive treatment with HAART immediately. As yet, no data show that treatment started early provides a better outcome, but supporters of early treatment argue several well-reasoned points. First, patients are healthier at this stage and therefore tolerate treatment better. Second, early in an HIV infection the virus may selectively infect and therefore deplete subsets of immune cells that are specific for the HIV virus. Therefore, aggressive early treatment with HAART may preserve these immune cells and allow the body to have a better defense against HIV. CDC guidelines recommend the treatment of patients in the acute phase.

The Asymptomatic Phase

The asymptomatic phase is perhaps a misnomer, as many patients have some chronic symptoms. In general, this phase includes persons with CD4 counts greater than 400 per mm^3, and few opportunistic infections or HIV-related problems occur. As CD4 counts drop between 400 and 200 per mm^3, patients have increasing symptoms of fatigue, fevers, night sweats, weight loss, and minor HIV-related difficulties, such as Candidiasis. As CD4 counts drop below 200 per mm^3, patients become effectively immunocompromised. CD4 counts decline by approximately 100 cells per mm^3 per year in an average patient with a modest viral load. This actually reflects the destruction of an almost inconceivable number of CD4 cells by the virus. Patients with high viral loads can progress faster, some progressing to below 200 CD4 cells per mm^3 in a year instead of the usual decade. A variety of factors have been identified that affect the progress of infection, including gender and race.[17]

The timing of HAART initiation has been a matter of some debate. The current International AIDS Society guidelines suggest that asymptomatic persons should begin treatment with HAART if their viral load is high (more than 55,000 copies per mm^3) and generally before their CD4 cell count falls below 200–350 per mm^3.[18] However, many exceptions to this exist. Debates rage over issues of clinicians' judgment whether patients are ready to accept treatment, whether they should start earlier or later, and what the best regimen will be. Much of the current controversy concerns whether certain medications should be reserved from early treatment in case a treatment-resistant virus develops, and another issue is the order of medications that patients should receive. There is a growing consensus that patients should receive the best possible treatment first, with the idea that this gives them the best chance of long-term suppression. The opposing argument maintains that they should receive medications that are sequenced so that if viral resistance develops, many alternative treatments will be available. The ideal approach to therapy still very much depends on the person.

AIDS

AIDS was previously defined by the first opportunistic infection, and persons developing any of the conditions in Table 1.2 are considered AIDS defined even if their CD4 count remains above 200 per mm^3. Once a person has a CD4 count below 200, he or she is now defined as having developed AIDS. This is the time when patients develop life-threatening opportunistic infections. HAART continues, but now patients receive prophylactic therapy and monitoring for known

Table 1.2. Indicator conditions in the case definition of AIDS (adults), 1997

Candidiasis of esophagus, trachea, bronchi, or lungs
Cervical cancer, invasive
Coccidioidomycosis, extrapulmonary
Cryptococcosis, extrapulmonary
Cryptosporidiosis with diarrhea longer than 1 month
CMV of any organ other than liver, spleen, or lymph nodes, such as the eye
Herpes simplex with mucocutaneous ulcer longer than 1 month or bronchitis, pneumonitis, esophagitis
Histoplasmosis, extrapulmonary
HIV-associated dementia: disabling cognitive and/or other dysfunction interfering with occupation or activities of daily living
HIV-associated wasting: involuntary weight loss greater than 10 percent of baseline plus chronic diarrhea (2 or more loose stools/day 30 days or longer) or chronic weakness and documented enigmatic fever 30 days or longer
Isoporosis with diarrhea longer than 1 month
Kaposi sarcoma in patient 60 years or over
Lymphoma, Burkitt immunoblastic primary CNS
Mycobacterium avium, disseminated
Mycobacterium tuberculosis, pulmonary, extrapulmonary
Pneumocystis carinii pneumonia
Pneumonia, recurrent-bacterial (2 or more episodes in 12 months)
Progressive multifocal leukoencephalopathy
Salmonella septicemia (nontyphoid), recurrent
Toxoplasmosis of internal organ
Wasting syndrome because of HIV (as defined: HIV-associated wasting)

Source: Data from Centers for Disease Control

opportunistic infections that are likely to occur. Effective prophylactic treatments for infections such as *Pneumocystis carinii* pneumonia continue to be important in persons with advanced disease. When CD4 counts are very low, typically below 50 per mm^3, patients also receive prophylaxis for *Mycobacterium avium-intracellulare* infection. In persons with less than 200 CD4 cells per mm^3, close monitoring is necessary for a variety of neurologic and psychiatric disorders.

Treatment

Only a few years ago, treatment for HIV was designed using a menu that had NRTIs in column A, NNRTIs in column B, and PIs in column C. The state of the art was generally considered two drugs from column A and one from column B or column C. This turned out to be a slightly oversimplified view, as several drug combinations were undesirable because of combined toxicity or the complication of dosing regimens (e.g., take pill B with food but take pills A and C on an empty stomach). Thus, the tables of regimens have grown longer and now list specific drug combinations by their degree of recommendation: recommended, not generally recommended but acceptable, and not recommended.

Table 1.3 shows the latest antiretroviral agents organized by class. For the most up-to-date combination recommendations, please visit the Johns Hopkins AIDS Service website at www.hopkins-aids.edu/guidelines/guidelines.html.

Psychiatry 101

A second purpose of this book is to present a basic method for thinking about psychiatry that is useful in rescuing the field from itself. In this view of psychiatry, psychiatrists are doctors, and not the rodeo clowns of medicine as they are portrayed on television and in the movies. It can be daunting to see psychiatrists in movies stalking their patients, and being stalked by their patients, as in *What About Bob?* With rare exceptions, psychiatrists are never the Marcus Welby type and are played by Mel Brooks rather than Mel Gibson. Even Barbra Streisand, as a sympathetic psychiatrist, sleeps with Nick Nolte in *The Prince of Tides.*

Sadly, it is not entirely fiction to present our field in a critical light. Psychiatry has some outrageous misuses for which to apologize, including the murder of mentally ill persons at the beginning of the Nazi holocaust, the sterilization of mentally ill persons in the United States, and the use of psychiatry in Russia to imprison political dissidents. More recently, we have brought the world alien abduction psychotherapy and past-life regression psychotherapy, and we are mired in a self-help and television-exposure culture extravaganza that mistakes platitudes for therapy.

Happily, psychiatry is rejoining the discipline of medicine slowly but surely

Table 1.3. Antiretroviral agents

Class	Agent, abbreviation (trade name)
NRTI	Abacavir, ABC (Ziagen)
	Didanosine, ddI (Videx, Videx EC)
	Emtricitabine, FTC (Emtriva)
	Lamivudine, 3TC (Epivir)
	Stavudine, d4T (Zerit)
	Zalcitabine, ddC (Hivid)
	Zidovudine, AZT, ZDV (Retrovir)
Nucleotide reverse transcriptase inhibitor (NtRTI)	Tenofovir disoproxil fumarate (Viread)
NNRTI	Delavirdine (Rescriptor)
	Efavirenz (Sustiva)
	Nevirapine (Viramune)
PI	Amprenavir (Agenerase)
	Atazanavir (Reyataz)
	Fosamprenavir (Lexiva)
	Indinavir (Crixivan)
	Lopinavir/Rotinavir (Kaletra)
	Nelfinavir (Viracept)
	Ritonavir (Norvir)
	Saquinavir hard gel capsule (Invirase)
	Saquinavir soft gel capsule (Fortovase)
	Tipranavir (Aptivus)
Fusion inhibitor	Enfurvitide, T-20 (Fuzeon)

through research, the illumination of mental illness, and self-examination. The view of psychiatry from Johns Hopkins has been long embodied in its psychiatric faculty and is covered in the book *The Perspectives of Psychiatry* by Paul McHugh and Philip Slavney.[19] We present a brief overview here.

Psychiatry is the discipline of medicine concerned with disorders of mental life. To deconstruct that definition a bit, psychiatry is a discipline of medicine. This means it must use the methodology of medicine to approach patients and mental disorders. Second, it is concerned with disorders, rather than simply any element of mental life. Last, it is concerned with mental life rather than just brain function. This definition is needed in part because of the enormous confusion and controversy surrounding the field of psychiatry.

The confusion in the field is partly because of the barriers in understanding mental functions and dysfunctions. Medicine moved from teaching students therapeutics in the 1800s to teaching diagnostics in the early 1900s. Psychiatry was firmly based in the medical tradition and attempted to follow suit. William Osler, considered by some to be the father of modern medicine, built on the established tradition of the bedside observation technique of Thomas Sydenham* in focusing on what was wrong with patients and organizing that understanding into disease categories, each with an etiology, pathophysiology, and a characteristic syndrome of signs and symptoms. He taught medicine at the bedside, focusing on the examination of patients, the knowledge base of medicine, and advocacy for patient care as fundamental to the art.

Psychiatry was sidetracked when neuropathologic study failed to disclose an understanding of most of the disorders in the field. Psychiatrists were stuck teaching therapeutics and, during the century that followed, made only modest progress toward rejoining medicine until these last decades. Almost all of the confusion and misadventures in psychiatric practice of the twentieth century can be traced to this problem. The problem of "dynamic" psychiatry fighting with "biological" psychiatry is essentially a fight over what type of treatment a patient will receive, without a discussion of what is wrong with the patient.

This book is organized around a series of psychiatric disorders that are categorized in a particular way. Some of the disorders, such as dementia, bipolar disorder, major depression, and schizophrenia, are presented as diseases. That is, they are syndromes and may be postulated to be a result of a structural or functional brain lesion. Other problems are not diseases but stem from other types of disordered functions. Some problems are the results of psychological insults from an experience in life. These problems, such as grief and demoralization, may cause a disorder just as profound as the previous ones, but are the result of the psychological effects of what a person encounters in life and do not involve any known lesion of the brain.

Some of the misunderstandings in psychiatry are because of the attempt to understand all problems in the field using one of these two methods. Throughout much of the twentieth century, psychiatry attempted to explain all disorders as a product of what a person encountered. The newborn can be seen as an unprogrammed computer, absolutely unmarred until life's "installations" begin to cause problems. This is what gave rise to ideas such as the schizophrenogenic mother: the idea that schizophrenia was the result of a particular kind of

---

*In the latter half of the seventeenth century, internal medicine took an entirely new turn in the work of one of its greatest figures, Thomas Sydenham, who has been called the English Hippocrates and the father of English medicine. He revived the Hippocratic methods of observations and experience. He was one of the principal founders of epidemiology, and his clinical reputation rests upon his firsthand accounts of gout, malarial fever, scarlatina, measles, dysentery, hysteria, and numerous other diseases. He introduced Cinchona bark into England and praised opium.

parental deprivation. The parents of some patients still wonder what they did to cause manic-depressive insanity in their child, just as family members wonder what they did to cause their child to develop diabetes. The difference is that endocrinologists do not write books entitled *The Diabetogenic Mother* and say that some parents have "a pancreatectomizing maternal style."

In the last two decades, psychiatry has recognized that some mental disorders are the products of diseases, much as Emil Kraepelin pointed out in the 1800s. The rediscovery of Kraepelin in the 1970s, which came about as efforts at Washington University in St. Louis strove to improve research on psychiatric disorders, ultimately resulted in the development of the *Diagnostic and Statistical Manual of Mental Disorders* (DSM), now in its fourth edition. The DSM began as an attempt to focus on those disorders in psychiatry that are diseases, clarifying many of the diagnostic considerations, and thus making diagnosis far more reliable by applying Kraepelin's disease logic to certain disorders of mental life.

The method Kraepelin used begins with the assumption that behind a syndrome is a lesion of a particular anatomical location or functional type caused by a specific pathological event. The lesion produces a set of deficits that occur in all patients. Pathoplastic features of the syndrome are determined by the ability of the person to compensate for the deficits, the requirements of the environment, and the severity of the lesion. The fundamental idea is that the deficits will be reliably seen across a group of affected individuals and be distinct from other conditions. This allows one to work toward identifying the etiology and pathophysiology of the disease. First one identifies the deficits. Then, using what is known about brain functions, one identifies an area of the brain that is likely to be associated with that impaired function. Then one examines the affected area for losses, looking for the lesion. Finally, the goal is to identify the areas of focal injury and determine the insult that caused them.

An elegant example is Parkinson's disease. James Parkinson identified a syndrome of visible motor dysfunctions that he described as the "shaking palsy." The symptoms included a slow, shuffling gait, a mask-like appearance of the face, tremors, and drooling. Some years later, Jean-Martin Charcot identified the syndrome in certain patients in his asylum and, based on physical examination, added the symptom of cogwheel-type rigidity, or stiff movements in the limbs that occur in short jerks as if driven by a cogwheel. He noted that, on autopsies, the patients had a loss of neurons in an area of the brain called the substantia nigra, which was not evident in patients without the syndrome. He renamed the illness "Parkinson's disease," and years later the importance of the neurotransmiter called dopamine from neurons in this area in the production of smooth movements was confirmed. Other neuronal damage to the same circuit, such as that in Huntington's disease, produces different but related motor disorders, yet these two diseases are readily distinguished by their different clinical appearance.

The DSM uses "operationalized criteria" to distinguish particular disorders. It has a tremendous strength in the reliability of a diagnosis when it is used to categorize diseases, but the DSM can be misused when attempting to create categories for disorders that are not diseases, such as the problems described in the following section. The DSM also runs the risk of being misused as a shortcut to a diagnosis, producing a profusion of algorithms, checklists, and screens that try to substitute for the traditional method of differential diagnosis used by doctors. Doctors in other disciplines do not rely on a checklist for a diagnosis. Instead they rely on a set of signs and symptoms that allow them to develop a differential diagnosis and a line of investigation for the confirmation of a final diagnosis. In much of this book, the clinical distinction between mental disorders will be presented as it would in most medical texts, directing attention to findings in the history and the exam that illuminate diagnostic decisions.

Four Categories of Disorder

The basic method of thought that underlies disease logic has been presented. The second category, disorders produced by one's life story or experience , is also familiar to most readers. These are disorders that lie in the psychological domain. Being raped can produce sexual difficulty later on, but it is unlikely that cells in the brain are specifically lesioned by the experience. A useful analogy is that a disease can be compared to a problem in the hardware of a computer, and problems of in one's life can be compared to problems in the software. X-rays, neuropathology, and electroencephalogram (EEG) studies may illuminate diseases, but they are unlikely to illuminate any facts in the case of a person who is angry about mistreatment during his or her formative years. Although experience is stored in the hardware of the brain, or the neuronal matrix, it is not grossly visible and needs to be read out as one might read out the programming code of a computer.

The psychological view of all psychiatric disturbances predominated most of the twentieth century. Although it was overused in psychiatry and was unable to provide much progress in the treatment for severe brain diseases, it did provide hope to all and a substantial benefit to many, so it should not be discarded in the myriad circumstances where it is useful.

The third category of psychiatric disorder contains those disorders produced by excessive or inadequate endowments. The "dimensional" traits of human beings are distributed in populations, frequently in normal or bell-shaped distributions such as the one shown in Chapter 4. Measurable endowments such as height, weight, appetite, sexual drive, intellectual endowment, and temperament can all produce states of vulnerability. Very tall people are more likely to bump their heads, survive nutritional deprivation less well, and are particularly vulnerable to injuries in falls. On the other hand, they can run faster and reach things on taller shelves in the kitchen. The selective or genetic pressures tend to favor those in the center of the curve, or the average, over long periods of time, although in a particular environment, everyone who is not at one extreme may suddenly find themselves at a significant disadvantage. For example, the average height for a man may produce the best survival over long periods, but in times of nutritional deprivation, the short may be better off, and in times of tall trees having the food, the tall may be naturally selected. Traits at the extremes of the curve produce people well adapted to a particular environment but vulnerable in other circumstances.

Problems of personality and intelligence fit into this category. Patients from extremes of the curve come to health care when their natural coping style fails in the face of the particular task they are confronting. Patients who are emotionally driven may do poorly when they face problems that must be addressed using "thinking" rather than "feeling" styles. Likewise, patients who rely heavily on cognitive approaches to life may be baffled and confounded by tasks that require emotional experience or expression. Emotionally overreactive patients often become stuck in behaviors that are destructive but are driven to their behavior by their feelings. Health care professionals, who tend to practice thinking rather than feeling styles, can find these patients incomprehensible. They are frustrated by the resilience with which patients return to doing things that are harmful to their lives. These kinds of disorders are discussed in Chapter 4.

The last category is that of motivated behaviors. Disorders of motivated behaviors are most familiar as addictions. Psychiatry, in the days of psychoanalysis, explained addictions as a product of one's life experience, while in the current DSM-based view psychiatry explains addictions as a disease. These disorders have special properties that distinguish them from the categories described above. Motivated behaviors have a biological basis and also are influenced by one's life story and personality, but they are distinct from life story problems, dimensional disorders, and diseases.

At the core of these disorders is the cycle shown and described in Chapter 5. Patients encounter an opportunity to engage in a certain behavior, and the completion of the behavior results in an activation of the internal brain reward system, leading to the desire to engage in the behavior again. Rewards of this type occur naturally for behaviors such as eating, sleeping, and sex. This positive feedback loop results in the amplification of desirable behaviors, and causes the development of a drive toward these behaviors that can maintain the behavior despite adverse experiences, and thus keep the organism, and species, alive. However, the cycle is subject to excessive amplification of other behaviors, such as alcohol or drug use, resulting in addiction. The number of different substance use disorder descriptions in DSM attempt to deal with the fact that these disorders evolve out of behaviors that are controlled and that the line between excess and disorder is not clear.

The current direction in the field of psychiatry is toward rejoining the field of medicine. The trend toward understanding psychiatry as a discipline of medicine, and toward defining a role for the psychiatrist as a doctor who specializes in disorders of mental life, will inevitably lead to better care for all patients. Beginning with a diagnostic formulation that distinguishes diseases of the brain from emotional reactions to life experiences is critical and will make the roles of different types of treatment obvious. The historical emphasis in this field on treatment specialization, as demonstrated by psychiatrists defining themselves as psychotherapists, group therapists, psychoanalysts, and, perhaps worst of all, psychopharmacologists, has been a source of much of the confusion in this field. No one in the field of medicine refers to themselves as a "nonsteroidal anti-inflammatorist." Medical doctors may specialize in the treatment of a particular type of problem, such as hematology, or in the treatment of groups of patients, such as pediatrics. In a hopeful trend, psychiatry is already developing new specializations around diagnostic categories, such as affective disorders or substance use disorder specialists, or specialization in particular patient types, such as child psychiatry or geriatric psychiatry.

The classification system for psychiatric conditions presented here will be used throughout this book to describe the types of psychiatric disorders that afflict persons with HIV, that are caused by HIV, and that complicate the treatment and prevention of HIV. Clinical examples of each type of problem are presented to clarify the principles of diagnosis and treatment. We hope that the reader will find the discussion and instruction enjoyable and informative, and that this book will inspire clinicians to intensify their efforts to help patients with these serious problems.

Case: Complicated Major Depression

A patient who we will refer to as A first came to the AIDS Psychiatry Service when she was 39 years old. She was referred by her primary doctor and a social worker in the HIV clinic. In addition to receiving medical care, she was being treated for polysubstance dependence in a methadone program. Although she was referred for presumed depression, she was in danger of being dropped from the substance abuse treatment program because of loud outbursts of temper, shouting at her drug counselor, and illicit drug use. Her counselor at the substance use program reported that there was something special about her, but she had used up all her chances and things seemed hopeless.

Throughout her childhood, A had violent outbursts and behavioral problems, including stealing, fighting, and lying. She performed poorly in school and was expelled from two schools for truancy and violence. She said that she had been "hyper" in school and that doctors had told her she was "hyperactive" but did not treat her. She quit school in the ninth grade when she became pregnant. She briefly held many service jobs, including work as a nurse's aide, but never had steady employment.

As a teenager, she began abusing both alcohol and heroin, and soon added cocaine. Her drug of choice became heroin; she was a daily injection heroin user throughout most of her adult life. She had been admitted to more than eight detoxification programs but never remained sober for longer than six months. She was arrested countless times and served three prison terms. At the time of her initial referral to the AIDS Psychiatry Service, she was unmarried and living with her aunt and her two children.

As well as asymptomatic HIV infection, with a CD4 count in the 700s per mm^3, A had significant chronic obstructive pulmonary disease and was unable to climb a single fight of stairs. She had a history of thrombophlebitis, subacute bacterial endocarditis, multiple pelvic infections, and a closed-head injury with a loss of consciousness. Her only medication was methadone, prescribed by her drug treatment program. In the past, mental health professionals in prison and at community mental health services had evaluated her and treated her briefly with psychological counseling and medications. She was uncertain what medications she had tried, but said that none of the treatments had helped her.

At our first examination, A was quite irritable, storming out of the room twice, only to return moments later. Sometimes she refused to speak; at other times she answered questions with an uncooperative, monotonal "yes" or "no." Her primary care doctor later described this as typical for her and said that she sometimes asked him for narcotics or benzodiazepines, but in an almost careless or insincere way. Upon initial evaluation, she complained only of extreme irritability. After a direct examination, however, she was found to have a sleep disturbance, with early wakening every morning; diurnal mood variation, with mornings worse than evenings; and a loss of pleasure in almost all the activities she had formerly enjoyed. She was essentially uncooperative with most of the exam, and she was incorrectly assumed to be cognitively limited based on the concreteness of her answers. She grudgingly promised not to commit suicide before her next appointment.

The team agreed on a provisional diagnosis of major depression, possible attention deficit disorder (ADD), and a personality disorder with mixed antisocial and borderline traits (Cluster B in the *Diagnostic and Statistical Manual of Mental Disorders, Fourth Edition* [DSM-IV]). She reported that she agreed to treatment only because of the threat of losing her place in the methadone treatment program and possibly her parole.

After a long discussion in the simplest terms (which she later said she found quite insulting) of the risks and benefits of treatment choices, A was prescribed desipramine. She promised not to use cocaine within seven days of taking desipramine. She showed a remarkable improvement on desipramine, after titrating to a dose of 225 mg/day. She became less irritable, she slept better, and her energy increased. She also reported better concentration and mood. For the first six months of treatment, all her caregivers remarked on her improvement, and she became much more engaged in treatment. She did well for about a year, but then began using drugs again and was dropped out of treatment after the death of a relative.

Three years later, at age 42, A was admitted to the hospital for the treatment of an episode of subacute bacterial endocarditis. The medical service inserted a Hickman catheter because of poor venous access, and intravenous antibiotics were started. Her first three hospital days were uneventful, but on the third hospital day she developed a fever after leaving the floor "to smoke a cigarette." A toxicology screen done with the fever work-up showed evidence of recent opiate use. When the infectious disease team attempted to discuss this with her, she insisted on signing out of the hospital against medical advice. Further, she refused removal of the Hickman catheter, insisting that the catheter belonged to her and she would use it to give herself intravenous antibiotics at home.

Because A seemed cognitively intact and had no evidence of either psychosis or a plan to harm herself or others, the infectious disease team felt obligated to discharge her. They feared, however, that she was at grave risk for severe sequelae from her endocarditis. Before discharging her, they requested a psychiatric opinion. When A was told that she could not leave until a psychiatrist saw her, she called the AIDS Psychiatry Service from her hospital bed and demanded to be seen immediately so she could go home.

The resident on the consultation service evaluated A. She determined that A was indeed a risk to herself, as her opiate cravings and impulsive nature made it impossible for her to resist using opiates, even while in the hospital with a life-threatening illness.

After the resident's evaluation, the infectious disease and psychiatry teams met with A to discuss a treatment plan. They told her that her endocarditis was life threatening and that she had a mental illness that impaired her ability to make decisions. They further told her that after she recovered, she could make decisions about her health care. The next time she was sick she could elect to be treated at another hospital, but for the acute phase of her endocarditis, which was at least five weeks, she would have to complete antibiotic treatment at Johns Hopkins. If necessary, she would be certified for involuntary medical treatment to ensure she received proper care. A was then offered a choice of finishing treatment on a locked psychiatric ward or staying on the medical ward if she agreed to a methadone taper, a restart of the desipramine therapy, and restriction to the ward until she no longer craved opiates (she had long since been discharged from her methadone treatment program).

A chose to remain on the medical ward. Her desipramine was restarted and she was tapered from opiates using methadone. She did extremely well and her endocarditis resolved. She chose to resume treatment at both the AIDS Psychiatry Service and the medical service.

After discharge, she kept her follow-up appointments. She received weekly supportive psychotherapy aimed at helping her learn to manage her intense feelings without acting on them. Her desipramine level was maintained in the therapeutic range, and her urine was routinely screened for drugs. She also rejoined her drug treatment program.

A was sober for seven years, with only two lapses. She continues to be seen by our team. She did well on desipramine, with trazodone and valproic acid added occasionally to control flares of her depressive illness. She requires oxygen for daily activities, and despite episodes of pulmonary edema and breathlessness, it took more than a year and a half to convince her to wear the oxygen apparatus regularly. She has a CD4 count in the 900s per mm^3 and no detectable viral load.

She has been intermittently employed, which has included caring for drug-addicted persons with AIDS. When she received her first-ever income tax refund, she brought the check to the clinic to show it to her therapist.

She recently had a severe relapse to heroin use after stopping her desipramine, but eventually was detoxified again and returned to her baseline state of the last eight years. She remains somewhat irritable and demanding, particularly when her depression recurs, but she works to control her temper because she now realizes that it impairs her effectiveness in dealing with the patients with whom she works. She has maintained a long-standing relationship with her therapist and psychiatrist.

Discussion

A illustrates the complex dynamics of many different psychiatric and medical problems overcome by the triumph of courage, fortitude, and even stubbornness. She was chosen as the first case for this book because she represents three things so well: the complexity of comorbid psychiatric disorders, the need for a clear diagnostic formulation to guide treatment, and, most important, the need for therapeutic optimism in the care of difficult and sometimes seemingly insurmountable psychiatric problems. The most important elements of her treatment cannot be derived from an algorithm; she could not be well described using the language of the DSM. One may, however, describe a comprehensive psychiatric formulation or a diagnostic impression using each of the four categories described in Chapter 1, and this will make appropriate treatment become clear.

A has the following disorders:

- Major Depression. Although not described in detail and not initially available, her family history supports this diagnosis. At her first examination she did not say she was sad, blue, or depressed and did not report a change in either her vital sense or self-attitude, but she did describe anhedonia and neurovegetative features of depression. More important, her problems are difficult to explain without a diagnosis of major depression.

- Substance abuse and dependence. This is an obvious diagnosis. It is important to recognize both A's addiction to heroin and cocaine, as they require different ways of thinking about treatment.

- Personality disorder. This patient has both emotional instability and extraversion. She is directed by feelings, what she wants and needs now, and by rewards, rather than by function and avoiding consequences. She is stubborn, emotional, and "difficult" by nature. These elements of her personality have directed much of the difficulty in her life.

- Life circumstances. The DSM uses the term *Adjustment Disorder*, which is woefully inadequate for this case. A has had a terrible life experience. Her trust and sense of how relationships operated were developed in an atmosphere of chaos without predictable rules. Intimate experiences were coercive, and she had no role models for relationships, commitments, and social development. She had little parenting. Her behaviors, driven out of temperament and circumstance, received random and unpredictable responses.

The first questions one might ask about treatment are "Why desipramine, rather than some other antidepressant?" and "Why not wait until the diagnosis of depression was more certain, because it was so unclear?"

Desipramine is a tricyclic antidepressant, with quinidine-like effects on cardiac conduction as well as other autonomic effects on cardiac function. This patient had a history of endocarditis and a history of cocaine abuse, both of which could make desipramine treatment more dangerous. Despite the danger inherent in its use, desipramine was likely to remedy the insomnia, irritability, and anhedonia associated with this patient's depression. It has additional therapeutic benefit in those with ADD (which A probably does not have, but seemed a likely diagnosis at the time). There is also some suggestion that desipramine might alleviate cocaine craving in some patients. (The data supporting desipramine's use for the treatment of ADD or to reduce cocaine craving are weak, but better than nothing.) The last reason to choose desipramine is the ability to monitor serum levels. It was explained to the patient that desipramine was dangerous unless used correctly, and this allowed us to measure whether she was taking it as prescribed.

As a psychotherapeutic maneuver, A was told how dangerous cocaine was in combination with desipramine. She was warned that it could easily give her a heart attack, and because at first she was thought to be possibly cognitively limited, she was told about it slowly and in detail. However, the major danger for this patient was that she would be expelled from her methadone program for using cocaine. Her counselor related that her next "dirty" urine would lead to certain discharge from the program. She seemed committed to her promise of not using cocaine.

It would be reasonable to argue that a safer way to treat A would have been to wait until the diagnosis was clearer, or to give an alternative antidepressant such as a selective serotonin reuptake inhibitor (SSRI). In the analysis at that time, however, the risks of desipramine with cocaine were less severe than the risks of getting back on street heroin, with the attendant risk of endocarditis.

It is also important not to discount the message embedded in the choice of treatment. "This is serious, dangerous medicine, because you have a serious, dangerous mental illness." Telling patients that they are mentally ill is not a trivial message. For some patients, it is worse than being told they have HIV or AIDS, and in our patients it comes in addition to being told they have HIV or AIDS. One patient said, "I would rather have cancer than a mental illness."

For A, the diagnosis of a serious mental illness is a double-edged sword. On one hand, she has HIV and now a mental illness. On the other hand, she now has some explanation for the difficulty she has had all her life. There is now a message of hope for change: "You are not a bad person; you are a sick person who can get better." The optimism contained in this idea cannot be overemphasized. It must, however, be deliberately exploited by the clinician. One cannot simply deliver the message that "you are mentally ill" without also saying, "and this is good news, because with treatment, your life can be your own and much better than it has been."

The other issue regarding this patient's mental illness is the necessity of placing responsibility on the patient for behavior. "You are sick, but your behavior, even if it is driven by mental illness, must change." This begins to address the patient's other disorders. An important issue for A is her impulsiveness, which is driven by her personality, her life experience, and her addiction. All of these elements needed to be addressed in her treatment.

It was frighteningly easy to predict A's relapse. Her relapse at one year involved the death of a family member, which led her to stop coming to the clinic for medications and to lose hope. There is no clear explanation why her second interaction with the Psychiatry Service had such a positive effect. One of the things she reported later was that even though she felt the team was mean to her, we were also the first people to see her as someone other than a "junkie," and this meant that we thought we could help her get well.

Many things should be discussed regarding this case. The depression has already been covered, and the treatment of depression is discussed extensively in Chapter 2. The issue of the treatment of personality disorder is discussed in Chapter 4, where we have described the vulnerability of some patients to an excessive focus on feelings and rewards. In this patient, we manipulated her behavior toward successful treatment by using rewards and positive reinforcement throughout her treatment. When she wanted forms filled out, such as those for housing, advocacy with agencies, such as calling insurers to get authorization for medical payments, and an endless stream of letters written to get her "entitlements," like disability and Section 8 housing, we insisted that she do something positive and measurable in terms of treatment in order to get those things from the team. As an example, she was required to come to four consecutive clinic visits and have negative toxicology screens before we would provide a letter supporting a move to more comfortable housing. Our directive was "attend certain meetings (that will be good for you), go to certain appointments (that will be good for you), and keep certain commitments (such as taking medicine that is good for you)."

The issue of the treatment of addictions is discussed in Chapter 5, and in this patient we focused first on groups, then on changing behaviors that were likely to provoke relapse, and finally on triggers for craving and lifelong habits that may have precipitated addiction in the first place.

The issues of psychotherapy are discussed in Chapter 7. In this element of her treatment we focus on the assumptive world, those things people expect and assume about the way to react to life and other people. In Chapter 7 we discuss issues of sexual misuse and mistrust and the way to recondition patients and improve coping skills to have a better response to adversity than they have had in the past. Overall, the way in which a coherent treatment plan for A, based on the combination of the principles in this book, aided in her recovery summarizes our work. Throughout her treatment, we focused on rewards rather than consequences, directed our efforts at her cognitive understanding of her goals rather than her feelings, and emphasized behavior rather than feeling. We focused on how well she had done rather than her setbacks, how much more she had rather than what she didn't have, and on the future instead of the present.

It is also important to discuss the ethics of our threat to admit her to the psychiatric ward involuntarily rather than allow her to leave the hospital against medical advice. Is it ethical to impose our view of health on another person? This gets at the core of the formulation. Her disorders are treatable, life-threatening conditions, and they impair her ability to make a decision about care that is rational and goal directed. She had a goal, but one that was driven entirely by feelings and the disorders of addiction, personality, depression, and life experience that she carried. This is an issue in the gray zone in medicine. On one hand, we have a commitment to autonomy, and on the other hand, a commitment to beneficence. The patient who wants an amputation because of the false belief that parasites have infested his arm would be injured by an emphasis on autonomy, whereas a Jehovah's witness who cannot accept a blood transfusion based on religious beliefs generally finds his wishes respected. The patient with delusions has impaired autonomy; his decisions are impaired by a brain disorder. A is similarly disordered. She is in the throes of an addiction, her views are colored by depression, her attention is focused on her feelings rather than her danger, and her experience with authority figures has left her with an impairment in the ability to form trusting and sustained relationships.

This patient's disorders remain difficult to treat. When we first saw her, she was an inarticulate, angry, irritable, and uncooperative woman. With treatment, she has blossomed into an articulate, angry, irritable, and somewhat more cooperative woman. When she is sick, the majority of her problem behaviors begin to resurface. What makes her so remarkable is the distance she has traveled in her journey toward being well.

In the course of this book, we will seek to persuade you that our patients have disorders that are understandable and remediable. With treatment, any patient might be able to get better. The problem is that not every patient will get better, but any patient might be the one. Because of this, we are obligated to try with every patient and hope that, like this patient, each can teach us to be better, clearer, more hopeful, and more effective in our roles.

Chapter Two
HIV and Major Depression

Depressive symptoms are the most common psychiatric complication of chronic medical illness. Studies have shown that depression has a negative effect on patients' adherence,[1] quality of life,[2,3] and treatment outcome.[4] Despite this important evidence, depressive conditions remain underrecognized, underdiagnosed, and undertreated in medical clinics.

Depression is a significant problem in HIV, as it serves as both a risk for perpetuating the epidemic[5-7] and a complication preventing the effective treatment of infected individuals. Persons with depression care less about their own safety, are hopeless, and are more impulsive. Moreover, HIV infection worsens depressive symptoms by creating an atmosphere of helplessness and stress. In an advanced infection, HIV creates direct injuries to subcortical regions of the brain. Fig. 2.1 may be viewed as a self-perpetuating cycle of increasing morbidity in a single patient or it may be viewed on a societal level, fueling the epidemic spread of HIV.

Differential Diagnosis of Depression

Disturbances of mood are common in HIV-infected patients, but they are often regarded as an expected result of problems associated with HIV or other aspects of patients' lives. The task of the clinician is to determine the correct diagnosis in order to apply effective treatments. Although many problems can result in complaints about mood changes, the most problematic issue is the distinction between a condition of major depression, which probably represents a disorder of the brain in which specific elements of the reward pathway and the centers that appreciate pleasure are disrupted, and the psychological reactive states of grief and sadness associated with loss or aversive experience. The term *major depression* is probably misleading, as grief, psychological trauma, and bereavement can be severe and produce a disorder or even suicide, but are probably

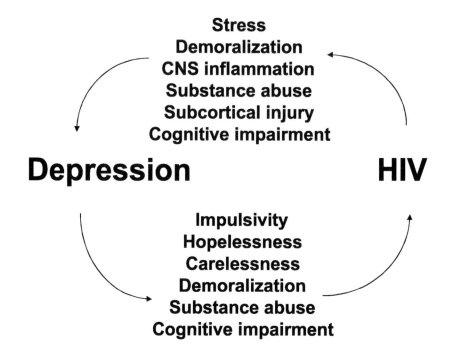

Fig. 2.1. A self-perpetuating cycle of increasing morbidity: depression and HIV

fundamentally different from major depression. The example of software problems as opposed to hardware problems in the computer is a useful analogy. Major depression represents a problem with the reward "chip" or "hardware" of the brain, whereas the psychological states of sadness related to loss represent a problem with the way in which a person has been "programmed" because of various experiences.

The differential diagnosis of depression includes states of grief and mourning (sometimes made quite severe by the person's vulnerabilities) and a variety of psychiatric syndromes that most likely represent disease states, including major depression (see Table 2.1). Patients with complaints of depressive syndromes can have dysthymia, dementia, delirium, demoralization, intoxication, withdrawal, central nervous system (CNS) injury or infection, acute medical illness, and a variety of other conditions. AIDS dementia and other HIV-related CNS conditions can produce a flat, apathetic state that is often misdiagnosed as depression. Cocaine withdrawal produces a depressive syndrome, and delirium can mimic many psychiatric conditions. CNS syphilis, a condition that had become quite

Table 2.1. Brief differential diagnosis of depressive symptoms

Depression (major depression and bipolar disease)
Demoralization
Dementia
Delirium

rare, has been reappearing in medical centers with HIV specialty services, and it remains "the great imitator," as it was called when it was originally described.

The diagnosis of major depression in an HIV clinic is complicated by the high frequency of depressive symptoms that are associated with chronic illness, significant losses and isolation, and complex medical treatments. The diagnosis may be further complicated by the presence of comorbid neurologic illness, comorbid substance use, and the use of many medications that can alter mental functions. Despite this, studies of patients with major depression have shown that their response to treatment is similar to that expected in other populations.

Whole books have been written on major depression, and even in uncomplicated patients the distinction between major depression and demoralization is not straightforward. We see major depression as a disease producing a set of deficits in the domain of one's affective life. The four primary elements of this domain are mood, vital sense, self-attitude, and hedonic responsiveness. Every person with depression has some constellation of symptoms within the matrix of these features.

Mood is the feature of affective life that describes the prevailing emotional tone a person experiences. Patients express depression as feeling blue, low, sad, or sometimes flat, devoid of emotion, or empty. Some say that they are miserable, in agony, anxious, worried, or angry, upset, and irritable. Although some are apathetic, most find the state extremely uncomfortable. Moods may vary with the time of day, usually worse in the morning and better in the afternoon, but sometimes in other patterns.

Vital sense is the subjective sense of well-being. Depressed patients say they are sick, have a heavy pressure in their chest, have low energy, and even feel themselves dying.

Self-attitude concerns the feeling directed toward one's self. Depressed patients feel guilty, that they are bad or evil, that they are undeserving of the things they have, or that they have failed those they love. (See Table 2.2.)

Pleasure (or a sense of reward) is associated with many behaviors of life, including those driven by appetite (such as sleeping, eating, and sex) and those associated with functions (such as work, hobbies, dress, social activities, and artistic expression). The suppression or absence of pleasure is a cardinal feature of depression.

Table 2.2. Depression

Depression diminishes:

- Mood: the sense of the baseline state of happiness that is usually present
- Vital sense: the sense of being well, healthy, energetic, alert, and able
- Self-attitude: the sense of being good, of doing well, of effectiveness, and of utility to others

Hedonic responsiveness refers to the enjoyment or positive reinforcement related to activities and experiences. This enjoyment can be divided into the rewarding aspect of pleasure and the satiation aspect. The reward might be termed the "Yeah" of excitement that one gets from an activity. An example is one of our patients who loves to bowl and experiences a surge of joy whenever he gets a strike. When he was sick with his depression, he said that bowling was boring. When he was well, he said that the "Yeah" was back when he got a strike. He said "Depression is a disease of your 'Yeah' receptors." The satiation element might be the "Ahhhh" of satisfaction after an activity. An example is the pleasure felt after one is very hungry and consumes a wonderful meal. Anhedonia describes the state in which hedonic responsiveness is blunted or absent, and is a principle feature of depression (see Table 2.3).

Neurovegetative symptoms are commonly associated with this syndrome. These include difficulties with sleep, appetite, concentration, and memory. Sleep disturbances can include insomnia or hypersomnia, but most often patients describe waking early in the morning with difficulty falling asleep again. Food intake and weight may be decreased or increased significantly, and patients often complain that food has lost its flavor. Appetite changes result in corresponding weight changes if untreated for long periods of time. Patients report slowed thought processes, with impairments in concentration, short-term memory, and occasionally generalized confusion. (See Table 2.4.)

The diagnosis of major depression in medically complicated patients is fundamentally difficult because of the sadness, loss, and demoralization that are the inevitable accompaniment of an illness. This means that patients undergo much sadness and a disturbance of their vital sense, even in the absence of major depression. In most HIV-infected persons, the diagnosis of major depression is easy, but in persons who have an advanced disease or who are ill, it can be difficult to decide if the person has major depression, demoralization, or both.

The presence of pervasive anhedonia pushes the diagnosis toward major depression. Persons with major depression do not become buoyed even when good things happen. One of our patients explained his lack of joy after winning the lottery was because of the inevitability that he would "just blow the money anyway."

Table 2.3. Anhedonia

Loss of reward (pleasure, satiation, or satisfaction) associated with behaviors:

- Appetite-directed behaviors
  - Sleeping
  - Eating
  - Sex
- Function-directed behaviors
  - Work
  - Hobbies
  - Exercise

Table 2.4. Disturbance of neurophysiology in depression

- Sleep
  - Early-morning awakening
  - Difficulty falling asleep
  - Disrupted sleep architecture
- Appetite
  - Change in food taste
  - Weight loss or gain
  - Immune function
- GI function

A second useful characteristic is that demoralized patients usually can be distracted from their sadness. When family comes to visit the patient in the hospital, most patients will enjoy the time and distraction until the family leaves, but patients with major depression will often say that they just could not wait until their family left, so they could be alone with their grief.

Somatic Symptoms of Major Depression and the Patient with HIV

Persons with major depression frequently present (most often to internists and family practitioners) with various and multiple somatic symptoms. These include, but are not limited to, headaches, gastrointestinal disturbances, inexplicable musculoskeletal or visceral pain, cardiac symptoms, dizziness, tinnitus, weakness, and anesthesia. Given the burdens of HIV, the medical problems associated with it, and the side effects of medications, depression may be very low on the list of considered causes of the patient's complaints. Even patients complaining of depressive symptoms may have overlooked depression or discounted it because of the presence of a plethora of other diagnoses.

Earlier in the epidemic, somatic symptoms of depression were commonly thought to be the result of HIV progression in persons with early-stage disease. In fact, nonspecific somatic symptoms are more likely to be the result of depression than HIV infection in persons who do not have another concurrent medical illness. In one important study, fatigue was found to be associated with depression and not HIV disease progression. The worsening of fatigue and insomnia at the six-month follow-up was highly correlated with worsening depression but not the CD4 count, the change in CD4 count, or disease progression (progress towards AIDS) by Centers for Disease Control (CDC) category.[8] This finding has been replicated in a longer study as well.[9] These findings support the notion that somatic symptoms generally suggestive of depression should trigger a full psychiatric evaluation.

In later-stage HIV infection, a variety of illnesses are common, moving depression down on the differential diagnosis list, closer to that potentially dangerous but sometimes appropriate label, the "diagnosis of exclusion." Somatic symptoms should always be evaluated carefully and considered in context (i.e., either with other indicators of the progression of HIV disease or with other indicators of depression). If somatic symptoms are misinterpreted, the diagnosis of major depression may be made too readily. In our experience, the problem has always been the underdiagnosis rather than the overdiagnosis of major depression, but the possibility of overdiagnosis remains. The significant danger inherent in overdiagnosis of depression is the potential to ignore other medical conditions that need treatment.

Some HIV-related medical conditions and medications can cause depressive symptoms. These include CNS disorders such as toxoplasmosis, cryptococcal meningitis, lymphoma, syphilis, and so on. Some investigators have found significant rates of depressive symptoms among male HIV patients with low serum testosterone levels.[10] Efavirenz, interferon alpha, metoclopramide, clonidine, propranolol, sulfonamides, anabolic and corticosteroids, muscle relaxants, cocaine, and many others have been reported to produce major depression or similar syndromes. Although these depressive syndromes often respond to withdrawal of the offending drug, when they do not, they should be treated as major depression with appropriate antidepressant medication. In particular, experience with the depressive syndromes caused by efavirenz and interferon alpha shows that treatment with antidepressant medications is well tolerated and often necessary for success.

In some special settings, the diagnosis of depression may be more subtle. The nursing home setting is notable for the fragility of advanced-stage AIDS patients with multiple medical illnesses and usually varying degrees of dementia. Serial observations by health care providers are most useful, as these debilitated or demented patients may not be able to clearly describe classic subjective symptoms of depression. Care providers will commonly encounter dysphoria (either sadness or irritability), apathy, decreased social interaction, negativism, sleep disturbance, and anorexia. Many patients with dementia develop behavioral disturbances, which may arise as catastrophic responses to unmanageable (even if minor) environmental provocations. Sometimes, however, behavioral disturbances are accompanied by a prominent and persistent mood disturbance indicating major depression. Because patients with dementia are very susceptible to delirium, it is crucial to distinguish that syndrome from an affective disorder.

Screening and Diagnostic Work-up for Depression

Routine screenings for psychiatric distress in patients at an HIV clinic can effectively preempt urgent referrals for rapidly progressing disorders. The combination of two brief, self-administered questionnaires, the Beck Depression Inventory (BDI) and the General Health Questionnaire (GHQ), can provide a simple and efficient screening tool. We validated these screening tests in a series of patients with a comprehensive psychiatric evaluation and found that a score of more than 14 on the BDI or more than 6 on the GHQ prospectively predicted a psychiatric disorder (other than substance abuse) with a sensitivity of 81 percent, a specificity of 61 percent, and a positive predictive value of 71 percent.[11] We recommend this screen (or an equivalent method) as part of the standard HIV medical clinic intake evaluation. All those patients who score above the screening thresholds can be referred to psychiatry for further evaluation.

Screening tests identify psychiatric symptoms and the likelihood of a psychiatric disorder, but they cannot make a diagnosis or distinguish various disorders from each other. Making a diagnosis of major depression requires a medical and psychiatric history and examination. A patient with a family history of depression, a history of the diagnosis of depression with successful treatment, and typical symptoms needs only a careful physical examination and a modest laboratory work-up before treatment. Blood count, simple chemistry to examine liver and kidney function, knowledge about CD4 cell count and viral load, hepatitis screening, and testosterone level may be the extent of the work-up. We usually screen thyroid function and check for syphilis as well. In older patients, patients with less typical symptoms, more compromised patients, or patients with medication-resistant depression, we would include the previous lab examinations and consider vitamin B_{12} level, the sedimentation rate, a spinal fluid examination, and brain imaging studies. Careful neurologic exams should be done in patients with an opportunistic infection history or low CD4 counts (less than 200 per mm^3).

Depression commonly exacerbates physiological symptoms and may in fact mimic them. It is critical, albeit most often difficult, to distinguish between depression presenting with prominent somatic symptoms and medical illness. Further, patients themselves will often misinterpret depressive symptoms and attribute low moods to the burden of having HIV, in essence making a layperson's diagnosis of adjustment disorder. The key to making the diagnosis of major depression in HIV patients is to follow standard psychiatric diagnostic practice, without overly discounting signs and symptoms either because of the putative severity of the stressors on the one hand or "organic" factors on the other. When depressive symptoms cluster together in the familiar syndrome, the diagnosis of major depression should be made.

Treatment of Major Depression

Pharmacologic Treatment

Pharmacotherapy is the mainstay of treatment for major depression. Several studies have demonstrated the efficacy of various antidepressant agents in HIV patients,[12-20] but to date no single antidepressant has been clearly shown to be superior in treating HIV-infected patients as a group. However, although all drugs may have equal *efficacy*, certain drugs may be more *effective* in individual patients. In large part, this may be because of patients' individual tolerances of certain side effects,[21] but the neurotransmitter profile affected by the specific agent may also play a role.

Aside from how well the pharmacology of the antidepressant matches a patient's disease, the engine that drives its effectiveness is patient adherence. Patients who reliably take adequate doses of antidepressants have the best chance of improvement. A general rule is to start at low doses of any medication, titrating up slowly to a full dose or therapeutic serum level (when meaningful) to minimize early side effects that may act as obstacles to adherence.

An algorithm for the stepwise pharmacologic treatment of depression is shown in Fig. 2.2. It is meant as a guide only, as thinking through all aspects of a particular case is the most fundamental way to choose the therapy.

Tables 2.5 through 2.7 list antidepressants, dosages, and common side effects. In many patients, the side-effect profiles of certain agents may be used to an advantage, and these "good-match" agents should be tried first. The next choices would be medications that do not have the type of side effects that would worsen

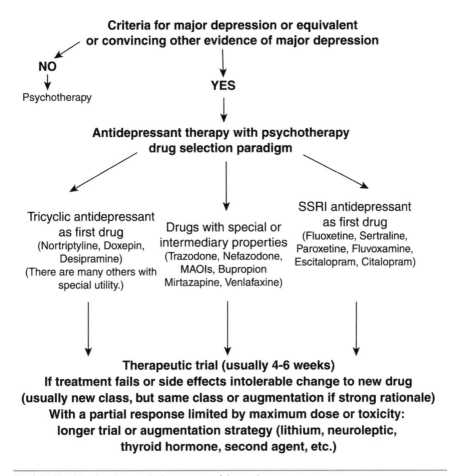

Fig. 2.2. Algorithm for pharmacologic treatment of depression

the patient's symptoms (e.g., a medication that is not associated with insomnia for a patient having difficulty falling asleep). Last resorts would include medications that have side-effect profiles that would likely exacerbate a patient's symptoms (e.g., a medication associated with increased GI motility for a patient with chronic diarrhea).

The first week of drug usage usually determines whether a patient will be able to tolerate the medication at all. Following this brief period, the dosage of any antidepressant should be increased slowly to either a typical full dose or a therapeutic serum level.[22-24] Once at this level, patients should be encouraged to wait as long as possible for the therapeutic effect, which may take longer than six

Table 2.5. Tricyclic antidepressant as a first drug (nortriptyline, desipramine, doxepin)

Property	Disadvantage	Advantage
Toxic and can be fatal in overdose	Suicidal patients	Allows insistence on drug screens and therapeutic blood levels
Quinidine-like effects on conduction and other cardiotoxicity	Dangerous when used with cocaine	Allows insistence on drug screens and therapeutic blood levels
Blood levels monitored for safety	Need for and cost of blood draws and labs	Monitors compliance and directs therapy
Anticholinergic	Dry mouth, constipation, urinary hesitancy, sexual dysfunction, sedation	Treats diarrhea, improves sleep
Antihistaminic	Sedation, weight gain	Improved sleep, improved appetite
REM suppression	Late-night REM with recalled nightmares	Decreased nightmares at initial sleep
Amelioration of chronic pain		Treatment of chronic pain, including neuropathy

Table 2.6. Selective serotonin reuptake inhibitor (SSRI) antidepressant as a first drug (fluoxetine, sertraline, paroxetine, fluvoxamine, citalopram, escitalopram, venlafaxine)

Property	Disadvantage	Advantage
Increased GI motility*	Diarrhea, nausea	Improved motility
Apathy*	Flattening of moods and drive	Diminished rumination
Delayed orgasm	Anorgasmia	Improved function in premature ejaculation
Minimal sedation*	Insomnia	No sedation
Large margin of safety		Safer in overdose and less toxicity

Note: There is some evidence that long-term use of SSRIs, particularly paroxetine (Fava M, Judge R, Hoog SL, et al. Fluoxetine versus sertraline and paroxetine in major depressive disorder: Changes in weight with long-term treatment. *Journal of Clinical Psychiatry* 61:863–67), can lead to modest weight gain, but in older patients after a stroke, fluoxetine was associated with weight loss (Robinson RG, Schultz SK, Castillo C, et al. Nortriptyline versus fluoxetine in the treatment of depression and in short-term recovery after stroke: A placebo-controlled, double-blind study. *American Journal of Psychiatry* 157:351–59).

*Not present or variable with some members of the class (see text)

weeks to achieve. Side effects should be assessed at every visit, and attempts should be made to treat any side effects the patient finds bothersome. For example, insomnia may respond well to subtherapeutic doses of trazodone (25 to 150 mg at bedtime). Constipation from a tricyclic antidepressant (TCA) often is relieved by increased water and fiber intake. Sexual side effects from selective

Table 2.7. Drugs with special or intermediary properties that might be chosen in special circumstances (trazodone, bupropion, mirtazapine, nefazodone, venlafaxine)

Drug	Disadvantage	Advantage
Trazodone	Needs a 400 to 600 mg dose to be an effective antidepressant	Very sedating, useful in refractory insomnia and depression
Bupropion	Lowers seizure threshold, activating (no sedation)	Little sexual side effects, no weight gain or sedation
Mirtazapine	Much weight gain, some patients get sedation	Some of the properties of tricyclics with less toxicity
Nefazodone	Sedation, potential hepatotoxicity, and drug interactions	Some of the properties of tricyclics with less toxicity
Venlafaxine	May have increased GI disturbance and may cause hypertension	Although mostly SSRI-like, less sedation and apathy are caused and efficacy in chronic pain

serotonin reuptake inhibitors (SSRIs) are common; impotence may be treated with sildenafil or other medications for erectile dysfunction in appropriate patients, whereas decreased libido and delayed orgasm may be alleviated by a drug holiday or by the addition of bupropion, buspirone, yohimbine, cyproheptadine, or ginkgo biloba.[25,26]

A gradual improvement in the depressive symptoms should be seen over the ensuing weeks of therapy. Rating scales—either formal, such as the Montgomery-Asberg Depression Rating Scale (MADRS), or informal, such as "rate your mood on a scale of 0 to 10, 0 being the lowest you've ever felt, 10 being the best"—are often helpful in determining progress. Patients who show only a partial response to a medication should be offered an augmentation strategy. The most common of these is the addition of a second antidepressant with a slightly different neuropharmacologic profile (e.g., adding venlafaxine or bupropion to an SSRI). Once again, the principle of "start low, go slow" applies.

Several other agents have been used to augment antidepressants. Although no trials for HIV patients have been published, the best studied of these is lithium,[27-30] but concerns about adverse effects often prevent primary practitioners from selecting it. Thyroid preparations, especially triiodothyronine, have also been shown to be of benefit[31,32] and may be of particular advantage to patients complaining of fatigue. Olanzapine[33] and ziprasidone[34] have also been reported to be effective augmenting agents, although many others have been used without support from the literature, including bupropion, lamotrigine, trazodone, methylphenidate, benzodiazepines, sleep deprivation, and bright light therapy, as well as other mood stabilizers and antipsychotic medications.

If no benefit is gained from the primary antidepressant, or if it must be abandoned because of intolerable side effects, a new primary agent should be chosen, titrated slowly, and augmented as necessary. Although drugs in the same class may produce similar side effects and therefore may not be tolerated, evidence suggests that a response may be seen from one drug where none was seen from another in the same class.[35]

Finally, clinicians often wonder about the interaction of antidepressant medications and highly active antiretroviral therapy (HAART) medications. The known interactions are listed in Table 2.8, but we must emphasize two points. First, because depression is associated with reductions in adherence to HAART, untreated depression may be as or more detrimental to disease progression than any medication interaction. Second, experience in working with comorbid HIV and depression has not yet shown clinical significance to drug-drug interactions (i.e., a need for dose adjustments for either antidepressants or HAART for successful outcomes).

Psychotherapeutic Treatment

At its most basic, psychotherapy is the treatment that changes the thoughts, feelings, and behaviors of patients through interactions with an expert. The process of change that occurs during psychotherapy may be described most simply as one that enables the patient to understand and develop active control over his or her actions, rather than *reacting* to his or her environment or acting without deliberation.

Psychotherapy is an important and integral part of treating major depression. It has been shown that medication plus psychotherapy is more effective for patients than either modality alone.[36] The difficulty arises, however, from the debate over the type of psychotherapy to provide. Among the individual psychotherapies, interpersonal psychotherapy and cognitive-behavioral psychotherapy are quite popular for treating depression. Although these modalities differ in their technical application, it has been difficult to show any difference in their outcomes. Jerome Frank has done some of the best work on comparing different psychotherapies and has showed that general improvements in demoralized patients treated with any structured form of psychotherapy did not differ in effect across modalities.[37]

The literature on the use of psychotherapy for treating depression in HIV patients is extensive, but clinical trial data are sparse. One study showed a significantly enhanced efficacy of either interpersonal psychotherapy or supportive psychotherapy with imipramine over cognitive-behavioral psychotherapy or supportive psychotherapy alone.[38] Improvements have been demonstrated as

Table 2.8. Interaction of antidepressants with HIV medicines

Drug	Starting dose	Usual therapeutic dose	Serum level	Advantages	Interactions with HIV medicines
Nortriptyline (Pamelor)	10–25 mg q hs	50–150 mg q hs	70–125 ng/dl	Promotes sleep, weight gain, decreases diarrhea	Increases nortriptyline levels: Fluconazole, Lopinavir/Ritonavir, Ritonavir
Desipramine (Norpramin)	10–25 mg q hs	50–200 mg q hs	More than 125 ng/dl	Promotes sleep, weight gain, decreases diarrhea	Increases desipramine levels: Lopinavir/Ritonavir, Ritonavir
Imipramine (Tofranil)	10–25 mg q hs	100–300 mg q hs	More than 225 ng/dl	Promotes sleep, weight gain, decreases diarrhea	Increases imipramine levels: Lopinavir/Ritonavir, Ritonavir
Amitriptyline (Elavil)	10–25 mg q hs	100–300 mg q hs	200–250 ng/dl	Promotes sleep, weight gain, decreases diarrhea	Increases amitriptyline levels: Lopinavir/Ritonavir, Ritonavir
Clomipramine (Anafranil)	25 mg q hs	100–200 mg q hs	150–400 ng/dl	Promotes sleep, weight gain, decreases diarrhea	Increases clomipramine levels: Lopinavir/Ritonavir, Ritonavir
Doxepin (Sinequan)	10–25 mg q hs	150–250 mg q hs	100–250 ng/dl	Promotes sleep, weight gain, decreases diarrhea	Increases doxepin levels: Lopinavir/Ritonavir, Ritonavir
Fluoxetine (Prozac)	10 mg q am	20 mg q am	Unclear	Activating	Increases HIV med levels: Amprenavir, Delarvidine, Efavirenz, Indinavir, Lopinavir/Ritonavir, Nelfinavir, Ritonavir, Saquinavir; decreases fluoxetine levels: Nevirapine
Sertraline (Zoloft)	25–50 mg q am	50–150 mg q am	Unclear		Increases sertraline levels: Lopinavir/Ritonavir, Ritonavir
Citalopram (Celexa)	20 mg q am	20–60 mg q am	Unclear		Increases citalopram levels: Lopinavir/Ritonavir, Ritonavir
Escitalopram (Lexapro)	10 mg q am	10 mg q am (per insert)	Unclear		No data
Paroxetine (Paxil)	10 mg q hs	20–40 mg q hs	Unclear	Somewhat sedating	Increases paroxetine levels: Lopinavir/Ritonavir, Ritonavir

(continued)

45

Table 2.8. (Continued)

Drug	Starting dose	Usual therapeutic dose	Serum level	Advantages	Interactions with HIV medicines
Fluvoxamine (Luvox)	50 mg q hs	150–250 mg q hs	Unclear	Somewhat sedating	Increases HIV med levels: Amprenavir, Delarvidine, Efavirenz, Indinavir, Loinavir/Ritonavir, Nelfinavir, Ritonavir, Saquinavir; decreases fluvoxamine levels: Nevirapine
Venlafaxine (Effexor)	37.5 mg q am	75–300 mg q am	Unclear		Increases venlafaxine levels: Lopinavir/Ritonavir, Ritonavir
Mirtazepine (Remeron)	7.5–15 mg qhs	15–45 mg q hs	Unclear	Promotes sleep, weight gain	
Nefazodone (Serzone)	50 mg BID	300–400 mg/d in divided doses	Unclear	Somewhat sedating	Increases HIV med levels: Efavirenz, Indinavir
Trazodone (Desyrel)	50–100 mg q hs	50–150 mg q hs for sleep; 200–600 mg q hs for depression	Unclear	Promotes sleep	Increases trazodone levels: Lopinavir/Ritonavir, Ritonavir
Bupropion (Wellbutrin)	100 mg q am	150–400 mg/d in divided doses	Unclear	Activating, no sexual side effects	

well for patients treated with group cognitive-behavioral therapy either as a single treatment modality[39] or combined with medication.[40]

In our clinic, we use a combination of cognitive-behavioral therapy and supportive psychotherapy for adjunctive treatment of patients with major depression. Cognitive-behavioral therapy seeks to help by asking patients to change their thoughts and actions at the direction of the therapist. In this form of treatment, therapists help patients identify particular ways of thinking or behaviors that exacerbate the depressive illness, and then patients are encouraged to develop thoughts and behaviors that promote health. An example of this is a treatment plan for a depressed patient that includes going to a day program or job every weekday to avoid the exacerbation of depression from lying in bed all day. The behavioral change on the patient's part leads to an improvement in mood symptoms over time and the reintegration into leading an active, healthy life.

Supportive psychotherapy is less directive and aims to help patients who are struggling with the disease aspect of their depression. These patients want to believe they can pull themselves out of depression, and they become frustrated when they continue to struggle with little results. They need education about the disease nature of their depression, encouragement to keep going, and therapeutic optimism that the treatments will work.

These therapies, applied judiciously and in combination with effective antidepressant medication, provide patients with a framework for the provider-patient relationship that is so crucial to success. The providers who keep the concept of psychotherapy in mind will structure the interactions with patients to slowly empower and enable the patients to control more and more aspects of their lives, thus relying on the providers less and less. This is in sharp contrast to the "consumer" or "client" role that has infiltrated the health care setting, in which patients choose the treatments they want, like a smorgasbord, with no direction by a treatment provider who is (a) there to provide expert diagnosis and a treatment plan based on evidence and a goal of successful rehabilitation, and (b) not impaired in judgment by depression as the patient is. Clients and consumers need to be converted into patients, and the principles of psychotherapy that we apply work well to accomplish this end.

Case: AIDS Dementia

B is a 37-year-old white single heterosexual male who was referred by a colleague in another city for evaluation of AIDS dementia and AIDS mania. He was initially seen with his parents and had advanced disease with almost no ability to function independently. He had recently been started on highly active antiretroviral therapy (HAART) but was only minimally compliant with his medications. He was living with his parents, who were afraid to leave him alone because he had set several fires inadvertently by leaving lit cigarettes on furniture. When unsupervised, he would search the house for alcoholic beverages, take things that belonged to others, and cause various damages. He had little or no recollection of these behaviors and seemed incapable of changing them. He required little sleep, talked constantly, and seemed unable to limit intrusive behaviors. He often refused his medications in a rage, yelled at his parents, and became embroiled in arguments over things that had not happened or that he had misinterpreted.

B had been an average to below-average student who was felt to be brighter than his academic performance suggested, but had attention difficulty and behavioral troubles. He had finished high school, graduated college with a marketing management degree, and worked in a variety of sales jobs. B had worked in his father's business but had quit because of his ongoing substance use and temper problems. He had also worked successfully for several other companies in related fields but had frequently been transferred from one location to another during his years of employment.

B had a long history of using alcohol, psychomotor stimulants, marijuana, and other substances, but it was unclear if he had ever been a daily user. It was clear, however, that his use had adversely affected his social, occupational, and family life. He denied intravenous drug use, homosexual contacts, or other HIV risk behaviors. The onset of his abrupt cognitive decline had triggered his HIV testing, and the result was a diagnosis of AIDS with 36 CD4 cells per mm^3 and a high viral load. He had a history of closed head trauma in a motor vehicle accident but had not lost consciousness. He had no other significant medical history. He had been diagnosed with attention deficit disorder (ADD) in childhood but had little formal psychiatric treatment. He had received substance abuse treatment at his parents' behest but had never remained in treatment, and he admitted that in the throes of his altered mood and circumstances he had given himself over to alcohol and was uncooperative with treatment efforts. B had seen several psychiatrists over the months before referral to the AIDS Psychiatry Service, but he had been uncooperative with their treatment efforts.

At the first evaluation, B was a pleasant, cachectic young man with a limited ability to attend to the examination. He was unable to perform simple cognitive tasks, partly because he was so distracted, and partly because he was cognitively impaired. He had rapid, forced speech that jumped from topic to topic. He rarely answered a question without strong redirection. At one point after he returned from using the bathroom, he was not sure if we had ever met, despite our having already spent more than an hour together.

He was euphoric, confident, and self-assured through most of the interview, smiling with satisfaction after completing long, rambling discourses that failed to answer simple questions. He smiled, assured the examining doctor that he was a great doctor, and expressed the belief that he (the patient) was going to be fine. When his mother began to weep after one of these reassurances, he ordered her loudly to stop crying. When told his behavior was unacceptable, he turned and smiled, apologized to his mother in what seemed to be a most contrite and genuine way, and then asked if that was an adequate apology.

He had occasional clear moments when he seemed to understand that he was seriously ill and needed help, but these were often quickly drowned out by a repetition of his litany of complaints about the care provided by his parents or by his confidence that things would be fine. He denied auditory hallucinations, obsessions, compulsions, phobias, or panic experiences. He described his mood as "outstanding" and did not feel sick or weak. He described himself as a good person who sometimes made it hard for his family. It was unclear whether it was fair to describe his belief that he would get well as a delusion.

He was unable to cooperate with any cognitive testing and was utterly unable to perform either a verbal or a written Trails B task, even though he was able, with lots of encouragement, to perform Trails A (essentially a connect-the-dots task). On the Folstein Mini-Mental State Exam, he scored 6 points out of a possible 30, but this seemed related to distraction rather than genuine disability.

Overall, he clearly had severe cognitive impairment consistent with advanced dementia. He had bilateral leg weakness with mild atrophy and complaints of some burning pain. He had a mildly decreased sensation in both legs that was worse at his feet. He had occasional slow, involuntary upper arm and facial movements, like slowed tics, which were described as somewhat choreiform.

B was given a diagnosis of AIDS dementia and AIDS mania. He was also given a diagnosis of polysubstance abuse. He was started on low-dose olanzapine and valproic acid (as Depakote). He was genuinely concerned when told he was likely to die and that he needed to cooperate with care, but he seemed earnestly committed to the idea of survival. Nursing home placement was also presented as a possibility to both B and his family. He was extremely resistant to this idea but did agree that if things did not rapidly change this would become a necessity. He agreed to take his medications exactly as prescribed as an alternative to being in a nursing home. He wrote himself several notes regarding this after being told of his memory deficit, telling himself why he needed to take medications, not to smoke when he was alone, and to follow directions.

His parents attended many sessions and learned about setting limits, creating distractions, and making physical changes to his environment. This included locking up all alcoholic beverages, removing all illicit drugs, and removing cues that could trigger problem behaviors, such as ashtrays, cigarettes, lighters, wine glasses, liquor glasses, and car keys. It became necessary to install locks on doors and certain closets in the home. His parents quickly caught on to the idea of distraction rather than argument. Instead of saying that he could not drive, they told B his car was in service or that he had lent it to a friend. They moved the alcohol from its customary cabinet and told him there was none. He was prescribed nicotine patches and was told that his father was bringing more cigarettes. He also had a series of notes he wrote to himself that his mother had him read, such as "Take the medicine or you will be locked up in a nursing home," or "Take the medicine or you will die."

Over the first month, B had only a slight improvement in his cognitive ability but rapid improvements in his behavior. His parents were initially quite skeptical, but they made a substantial effort to cooperate with his treatment. B also had a precipitous decline in his hyperverbal state and became more concerned about his illness as his general elevated mood and distractibility faded.

He came for monthly appointments and, as his deficits improved, he became increasingly aware of his deficits and the gravity of his situation. He began to attend substance abuse group meetings, began wearing a crucifix, and was much more forthcoming about his behaviors. He remained sober and continued to take his medications reliably. His viral load fell to undetectable levels and his CD4 cell counts came up to the 300s per mm^3. His cognition slowly improved over the next year, yet he continued to have considerable difficulty and bilateral leg weakness with mild atrophy. He eventually was able to start part-time work, but often became tearful with frustration over his cognitive deficits. Olanzapine was tapered uneventfully and he continued to improve.

Approximately one year into his course, his family reported that he had become more withdrawn, somewhat tearful, and much more irritable. He was prescribed low-dose paroxetine and underwent an almost immediate improvement in his mood and attention. Over the next several months, he started a relationship with an HIV-uninfected woman and came for counseling with her before initiating a sexual relationship with her. She called at various times to report that his mood was depressed or euphoric, that he was more or less irritable, or that he was more or less withdrawn. He had no recurrence of his manic symptoms at any time, and he complained of sedation with the Depakote, which was tapered after about 18 months. B also experienced mild episodes of depression that promptly improved with adjustments of paroxetine, and he had continued insomnia that responded to occasional treatment with trazodone.

As of this writing, B has married his girlfriend, works full time, and successfully passed a licensing examination for a change in profession. He retains about 90 percent of his baseline cognition, remains sober, and sees his recovery as the miracle that it is, as does his family.

Discussion

This case illustrates the principal problem of treating AIDS dementia. Patients with apathy do not bother to take medications, and those with mania refuse to do so, often believing they are already cured. Few have the resources to be flown to a tertiary care center or have parents who will devote themselves full time to their care for the months required to recover. Even with all of these assets, some patients return to drug-using behavior or alienate caregivers as soon as they begin to recover. Nonetheless, B had a dramatic response, mostly owing to his own willingness to appreciate and treasure his miraculous recovery and to his family's devotion and commitment. It also helped that he received medical care from an outstanding HIV doctor.

Before the advent of HAART, such patients received high-dose AZT, sometimes more than 2 grams a day, as tolerated by the patient and his or her hematopoietic system. Even in this setting, some patients had dramatic results. The problem was getting adequate resources for the patient to receive medication daily. Nursing homes have extensive experience with this problem but frequently are ill equipped to care for patients with mania who are up all night, hyperverbal, and often quite strong and therefore capable of meaningful resistance even when not competent. Outcomes for patients with advanced dementia are unpredictable and can be far better than expected, provided they are fortunate enough to be able to benefit from the treatments that exist.

It would be easy to say that B recovered on the strength of his resources, but similar miracles occur for patients with fewer resources, and patients with similar resources often fail treatment. AIDS dementia is probably currently the single most lethal HIV-associated condition because it destroys the opportunity for patients to understand the situation and cooperate with their care providers. Occasionally, despite the depredations of the illness, we see a patient like B, who remains an inspiration to anyone trying to recover from the true loss of one's mind.

Chapter Three
Other Psychiatric Diseases in the HIV Clinic

Several psychiatric diseases are encountered frequently in the HIV clinic. Little epidemiological data exists to prove that these conditions directly promote HIV infection, but ample evidence shows that they are associated with risky behaviors, a decreased quality of life, and barriers to good medical care. Chronic mental illnesses such as schizophrenia, bipolar disease, and the conditions associated with impaired cognition (including AIDS dementia, mental retardation, and even HIV minor cognitive-motor disorder) all influence behaviors that transmit HIV and other diseases. They also have an effect on the way medical care providers perceive their patients and the amount of resources that patient care consumes. Although the overall prevalence of these diseases involves many thousands of fewer patients, the effect of the diseases themselves is profoundly devastating to the individuals whom they afflict. In this chapter, we will discuss the diseases that primarily affect cognition: delirium, AIDS dementia, minor cognitive-motor disorder, bipolar disorder (manic depression), schizophrenia, and some anxiety disorders.

Delirium

No book on the mental difficulties associated with HIV is complete without a discussion of delirium. This diagnosis has engendered much confusion and may be a source of friction among psychiatric consultants and primary medical teams. Delirium has also been called diffuse encephalopathy, a term emphasizing the global nature of brain dysfunction associated with this state. Some of the best investigation into the causes and outcomes of delirium comes from work in geriatric populations, as elderly people are at a higher risk for delirium than younger adults.

One very well conceived model has been published by Inouye and colleagues, and it holds that most delirium is likely a "two-hit" phenomenon, meaning that patients are made vulnerable when they are frail, and then suffer some acute precipitant that pushes them over the edge to delirium. Certain predisposing factors increase the likelihood of delirium in an individual, and this likelihood increases as the number of predisposing factors increases. Further, certain precipitating factors can lead to delirium in any patient, but less severe precipitants can bring about delirium in a highly predisposed individual.[1]

Although this model has not been replicated in HIV-infected individuals, it has face validity. The predisposing factors for elderly patients include items such as the severity of the disease burden and sensory deficits (which would impair an individual's ability to self-reorient). Similar conditions can be found in HIV patients, such as inanition, central nervous system (CNS) damage, and visual loss from *Cytomegalovirus* (CMV) retinitis. The precipitating factors in the elderly include new medications, new medical problems leading to decreased mobility, less reorienting interaction with the outside world, and malnutrition. For HIV patients, precipitants might be new medications, new opportunistic infections, or hospitalization.

Delirium is the result of a diffuse brain dysfunction that occurs acutely or subacutely. It is easily appreciated by studying intoxication states, including those caused by medications and illicit drugs; withdrawal states, such as delirium tremens (DTs); and metabolic disturbances, such as hypoxemia and electrolyte imbalance. Delirium is not the result of a single specific lesion, but a general description of a state of widespread disarray of many brain functions.

Textbooks emphasize three elements in defining delirium: a disturbance of the level of consciousness (with patients ranging from hypervigilant to sedated and stuporous), an impairment in the ability to direct and maintain attention (with distractibility and a difficulty to focus and interpret), and the waxing and waning nature of delirium (patients will seem better at some times and worse at others). Patients will also be confused and have difficulty with memory and cognition (patients are often amnesic about events that occur during delirious states). In addition, they may demonstrate erratic emotional states and often have impaired judgment.

Delirium has been shown to lead to poor outcomes, as it generally occurs in severely ill patients, but it is also often missed by physicians, particularly in cases where other psychiatric conditions are also present. As an example, a clinician would seldom overlook a patient with DTs and hallucinations, but when the patient also has schizophrenia, the hallucinations may be attributed to that diagnosis and therefore be misdiagnosed.

Some common causes of delirium are the various intoxication syndromes associated with medications and intoxicants. Medicines that block acetylcholine receptors in the brain, the so-called muscarinic receptors, are particularly implicated. These types of anticholinergic delirium are so common that the medication physostigmine, which increases acetylcholine at receptors, was given the trade name "Antilerium" and was often injected into hospitalized patients suffering from delirium at the bedside, sometimes with dramatic results. Many drugs, even those readily available over the counter, have an anticholinergic effect,[2] and those with sedating and antihistamine properties are frequent culprits. Narcotic pain medications, sedative-hypnotic medications, particularly benzodiazepines, and general anaesthetic agents also are common causes of intoxication-type delirium. Theophylline, digoxin, corticosteroids, antidepressants, mood stabilizers, and antipsychotics may cause delirium. Illicit drugs are sought by some individuals for their intoxicating effects; those same effects may cause prolonged delirium in a predisposed host.

A variety of medical conditions can precipitate delirium in a vulnerable patient. Hypoxemia, hyponatremia, hypercalcemia, an inadequate brain perfusion from any cause (usually low blood pressure), seizure activity, sepsis, and a great number of other medical problems may profoundly impair cognitive function and consciousness. A CNS infection may be present with delirium in immunocompromised patients and may be the only sign of infection. Intensive care unit (ICU) psychosis, a common term for delirium associated with the ICU, demonstrates the results of combining sensory deprivation with a compromised medical condition and is a form of delirium that can have tragic results. Withdrawal from alcohol, benzodiazepines, and barbiturates (or related compounds) causes DTs, which can be fatal if unrecognized and untreated. The abrupt withdrawal of steroids in a steroid-dependent patient may precipitate an Addisonian crisis, a medical emergency related to the abrupt loss of glucocorticoid in the bloodstream, with possible attendant delirium.

The treatment of delirium centers around three major efforts. The first is the identification and treatment/removal of the underlying causes or precipitating factors. The patient must be carefully examined and any abnormal findings investigated. Careful history-taking is paramount, and the chronology of changes in medications or medical status is very important, because it often lends a clue to the precipitants.

The second effort is reorientation and environmental regulation. Delirious patients should be reoriented regularly. Because sensory deprivation is disorienting, patients should be allowed access to reorienting stimuli, such as windows, television sets, calendars, and clocks. The personnel caring for the patient should reintroduce themselves regularly and frequently remind the patient of the time and place. Room lights should be on in the daytime and off at night. Often, psychiatric wards and nursing homes are model environments for the care of delirious patients, because the community or milieu is more orienting than general medical wards. In psychiatric wards or nursing homes, patients are out of bed and in a common area during the day; they take meals in a dining room and interact with other people. Hospital wards, however, generally have patients in beds, either alone or with a single roommate, with a more limited range of interactions and thus fewer reorientation opportunities.

Finally, the treatment of delirium includes sedation if the patient is potentially violent or could cause injuries to him- or herself because of poor judgment. Restraint may be used but should be done with caution and for a short duration, as it leads to more disorientation because it limits one's ability to move around and acquaint one's self with the immediate surroundings. In general, we favor low doses of high-potency antipsychotic agents or atypical antipsychotic medications for calming agitated patients. Benzodiazepines should be considered for patients in alcohol or benzodiazepine withdrawal, and can be used to sedate delirious patients, but may worsen the delirium and cause behavioral disinhibition.

AIDS Dementia

Shortly after the first cases of AIDS were recognized, patients presented with a variety of devastating brain lesions and cognitive deficits. Early in the epidemic, a group of patients were identified as having a rapidly progressive dementia syndrome. Initially, the search for infectious etiologies to explain these symptoms was a major research effort. Many CNS opportunistic infections and conditions related to immunosuppression were identified. These included progressive multifocal leukoencephalopathy (PML) and cytomegalovirus encephalitis (viral diseases), cerebral toxoplasmosis (a parasitic infestation), cryptococcal meningitis (a fungal infection), and CNS lymphoma (a neoplasm). Further, immunosuppressed patients presented with a higher incidence of herpes encephalitis, tertiary syphilis, and intracerebral vasculitis. The first, specific HIV-induced neuropsychiatric disorder identified was the AIDS dementia complex.

Patients with AIDS dementia present with slow cognitive functioning. The tasks that are affected are those accomplished using structures referred to as the subcortical areas of the brain, where information is routed and moved. In particular, the basal ganglia[3] and nigrostriatal[4] regions appear to be the most damaged. Other dementias, such as Alzheimer disease, primarily affect the cortical neurons and cause a loss of information stored there, such as specific memories of names, words, and associations. Early in Alzheimer disease, patients have difficulty with the names of objects, get lost, and cannot remember things. In AIDS dementia, as in other subcortical dementias such as Parkinson and Huntington diseases, the ability to access and manipulate information in particular ways, sometimes described as psychomotor speed, is affected earliest and most profoundly. Patients' performance with the grooved pegboard, the Hopkins Verbal Learning task, and the Trailmaking B task are affected earlier and more severely by AIDS dementia than in the memory and recall tasks that identify patients with Alzheimer dementia.[5] Abnormalities using the grooved pegboard task have been directly correlated with subcortical neuropathology on magnetic resonance imaging in HIV patients.[6]

The relationship between AIDS dementia and other subcortical dementia syndromes such as Parkinson's and Huntington's diseases is further reflected in the high rate of Parkinsonian symptoms seen in AIDS dementia patients,[7] who may be further worsened by treatment with dopamine blockers[8] or opportunistic infections.[9]

An early diagnosis is best accomplished by careful examination, but it can be aided by screening using short bedside tests. The verbal Trailmaking B test seems quite sensitive but has limited specificity. A poor performance on this task should lead to a thorough evaluation. In this test, the patient is asked to say the alphabet, then to count in sequence, and finally to combine the alphabet with the corresponding number in sequence, starting with a-1, b-2, c-3, and so on. Mistakes include skipping a number or letter in the sequence (a-1, b-2, c-3, d-5) or maintaining one number or letter continually (a-1, b-2, c-3, d-4, d-5, d-6), called *perseveration*. Patients with a variety of conditions perform this task poorly, but AIDS dementia patients will often have difficulty with this task even after having a relatively good performance on other tasks and very early in their course before their condition is otherwise clinically apparent. A bedside AIDS dementia screening test has been developed at Johns Hopkins by Justin McArthur's group and is useful in both making a diagnosis and for tracking progression (see Exhibit 3.1).[10]

As in other subcortical dementias, patients with AIDS dementia develop symptoms within the subcortical triad of memory, mood, and movement (the three M's), otherwise known as dementia, depression, and dyskinesia (the three D's). Memory loss usually comes first, but on some occasions affective symptoms, especially apathy, may precede it. As the condition advances, patients often demonstrate an apathetic state of emotional indifference. They may also develop a mood disorder, either classic major depression with pervasive sadness, distress, and hopelessness, or mania, as described later. Either apathy alone or concomitant sadness and hopelessness may lead patients to poor self-care, inattention to their surroundings, and loss of social functions. The most devastating feature may

Exhibit 3.1. HIV dementia screening test

Score	*Maximum*	
( )		Memory—Registration

Give the patient four words to recall (dog, hat, green, peach) with one second to say each. Then ask the patient all four words after you have said them.

( )	6	Psychomotor Speed

Ask the patient to write the alphabet in uppercase letters horizontally. Record the time in seconds.

Less than 21 sec. = 6; 21.1–24 sec. = 5; 24.1–27 sec. = 4; 27.1–30 sec. = 3; 30.1–33 sec. = 2; 33.1–36 sec. = 1; more than 36 sec. = 0

( )	2	Constructional

Ask the patient to copy the 3-D cube below. Record the time in seconds.

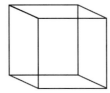

Less than 25 sec. = 2; 25–35 sec. = 1; more than 35 sec. = 0

Source: Davis HF, Skolasky RL, Jr., Selnes OA, Burgess DM, and McArthur JC. Assessing HIV-associated dementia: Modified HIV dementia scale versus the grooved pegboard. *AIDS Read* 12(1): 28, 29, 31.

be the loss of interest in or even the capacity to take highly active antiretroviral therapy (HAART). This is particularly problematic, as HAART has some degree of effectiveness in slowing, and in some cases reversing, the dementia process.[11]

If possible, conduct this test in a quiet environment. Establish rapport with the patient and praise good effort, regardless of success. The instructions for each section of the test are as follows and are also listed in the exhibit itself:

- Memory registration. Tell the patient you would like to test his or her memory. "I am going to ask you to remember four words. These are the words: dog, hat, green, peach." Speak the words clearly and slowly, about one per second. Ask the patient to repeat the words. If the patient does not remember the words, repeat all the words (not just the one[s] the patient did not recall) until the patient can repeat all of them. If the patient cannot register the words after five trials, recall cannot be meaningfully tested. The registration part of the test is not scored.

- Speed of processing. Provide the patient with a blank sheet of paper in the horizontal position and instruct the patient to write the letters of the alphabet (uppercase) with a ballpoint pen as quickly as possible. Measure the time in seconds to complete the task. If it is unclear whether the patient is sufficiently familiar with the alphabet to perform the test, ask the patient to recite the alphabet. If the patient is unable to do so, ask the patient to write the numbers from 1 to 26 instead, and time this. Convert the score in seconds to a point value.

■ Visuoconstructional abilities. Provide the patient with a model of a three-dimensional cube and ask the patient to copy it as quickly and as accurately as possible. Time this in seconds using a stopwatch. Convert the raw score to a point value.

■ Recall of four words. After approximately three to five minutes, ask the patient to recall the four words. Give one point for each word spontaneously recalled. For words not recalled, prompt the patient with a semantic cue as follows: animal (dog), piece of clothing (hat), color (green), and fruit (peach). Score a half-point for each word correctly recalled after prompting. A score of less than seven is considered abnormal.

AIDS dementia is complicated in many patients by the development of agitation, insomnia, irritability, and in some cases euphoria and psychosis. This condition has been termed AIDS mania and significantly complicates the treatment of dementia. Patients are often unwilling to take medication, as they may believe themselves to be well or cured, or are simply uncooperative. Such patients are difficult to manage because of their increased agitation, talkativeness, insomnia, and irritability. They require increased resources and often need institutional care. Treatment for such patients is described in the section on bipolar disorder, and although few data exist, experience shows that this condition improves with HAART[12] and psychotropic medications.

Most cases of AIDS dementia are associated with movement disorders, especially gait disturbances and fine motor deficits. Occasionally, patients will present with acute dystonia. Motor symptoms may be subtle in early stages, including occasional stumbling while walking or running, the slowing of fine repetitive movements, such as playing the piano or typing, and slight tremors. On examination, patients will demonstrate impaired saccadic eye movements, dysdiadochokinesia, hyperreflexia, and, especially in later cases, frontal release signs (grasp, root, snout, and glabellar reflexes). In late stages, the motor symptoms may be quite severe, with marked difficulties in smooth limb movements, especially in the lower extremities. Impairments during psychomotor speed tests by patients with no memory complaints at the time of an AIDS diagnosis have been shown to predict the development of HIV-associated dementia up to two years prior to its onset.[13]

Although the clinical description of the syndrome has become fairly well refined and widely recognized, research has not fully elucidated the mechanisms of the disease process. As stated, the primary structures affected in AIDS dementia are the basal ganglia and nigrostriatal pathways, followed by diffuse neuronal loss. The pathophysiology likely involves macrophage and migroglial activation and the release of cytokines, metalloproteinases, and chemokines that cause neuronal dysfunction and demise.[14,15] Further, viral products Tat and gp120, along with tumor necrosis factor-a (TNF-a) released from macrophages may also cause neuronal death.[16,17] AIDS dementia is often a disease that affects patients in the late stages of AIDS, with high viral loads and low CD4 counts. As HAART has helped reduce the amount of time patients spend with an advanced illness, HAART has significantly decreased the incidence of AIDS dementia.[18,19]

Neuroimaging studies have revealed significant white matter changes in late-stage AIDS dementia that improve with a successful HAART treatment.[20] Immunohistochemical studies have shown high densities of HIV viral antigen in regions suggested as foci for disease by imaging studies, including caudate[21] and globus pallidus.[22] Functional MRI studies have shown an increase in brain activation during working memory tasks in patients with known cognitive deficits[23] and in HIV-infected patients that later developed cognitive deficits.[24] The overall message for these studies is that high densities of a virus as well as low CD4 counts predict the development of AIDS dementia. Also, pathophysiology of AIDS dementia is multifactorial, including HIV and cytokine factors related to the damage of neuronal and glial cell destruction.

As unfortunately occurs in medicine, advances in treatment development far exceed the realities of treatment implementation. HAART dramatically alters the course of AIDS dementia in many patients, either stopping the progress or in some cases reversing the dementia. However, these same patients pose the greatest challenge with regards to adherence and outcome. The dementia decreases health care providers' ability to assess patients and affects the patients' ability to attend clinics. Dementia also impairs patients' ability to reliably remember to take medications, take them correctly, and report medication adherence. Apathy accompanies all subcortical disruptions and makes it less likely that patients will take their medication. Apathy is not necessarily major depression, but it may be an independent, uncaring, emotionally disconnected state of being. Affective disorders in patients with AIDS dementia, namely major depression and AIDS mania, contribute significantly to medication nonadherence.

At present, HAART is the mainstay of treatment for AIDS dementia. Certain antiretrovirals penetrate the CNS in higher concentration, and open-label trial results have shown an improvement in neuropsychological testing for patients treated with AZT (Zidovudine, Retrovir).[25] This initially made CNS-penetrating drugs a favored choice in the treatment of patients with AIDS dementia. Studies that have examined outcomes suggest that many HAART regimens correlate with clinical improvements in dementia[26-28] and improvements in brain metabolite abnormalities[29,30] and neurotoxin suppression.[31] Our standard of care is to choose the best possible HAART regimen for the patient based on clinical indicators.

As stated previously, however, the major impediment is patient adherence. The addition of low-dose stimulants such as methylphenidate can be helpful to relieve apathy in patients with AIDS or other subcortical dementia,[32,33] but it may not be enough to get patients to take their medications reliably. Many patients, especially those with advancing dementia, will benefit from medication monitoring that can be supplied in a skilled nursing, assisted-living home or a family supervision setting. Currently no data support the use of cholinesterase inhibitors to slow the progression of AIDS dementia.

Minor Cognitive-Motor Disorder

Although AIDS dementia is diagnosed in patients with CD4 nadirs less than 200 cells per mm³, a less severe neurocognitive disorder emerges in earlier HIV infections known as minor cognitive-motor disorder (MCMD) or mild neurocognitive disorder. The symptoms of MCMD may be very subtle and are essentially mild manifestations of the same symptoms seen in AIDS dementia: cognitive and motor slowing. Often, the disorder is discovered as a result of a patient's specific minor complaint, such as taking longer to read the newspaper, experiencing dysfunction when performing fine motor tasks (e.g., playing the piano), an increased tendency to stumble or trip, or finding mistakes when balancing the checkbook. The disorder is confirmed when mild impairments are present in at least two of the following domains: verbal/language, attention, memory (recall or new learning), abstraction, and motor skills.

Prevalence data for MCMD are variable, with up to 60 percent prevalence by the time of AIDS definition. Prevalence in earlier stages is not well defined, but the disorder has been anecdotally reported preceding a diagnosis of AIDS by 11 years.[34] Whether MCMD predisposes to AIDS dementia is also of some debate. It appears that some patients may continue to have minor problems, whereas another group will progress to frank dementia.

With regard to treatment, no controlled data are available. HAART may be of some benefit in slowing progression, but this conclusion is confounded by a lack of understanding the factors that lead some patients to progress while others remain static.

Bipolar Disorder (Manic-Depressive Disorder)

Bipolar disorder is a disease that affects the affective domain of one's mental health. A patient's emotions become disconnected with his or her environment and may be "stuck" in either a depressive mode, similar to the syndrome presented in the last chapter, in an expansive or elevated mode, or some combination, referred to as a mixed state. In the classic descriptions of manic-depressive illness, patients spend periods of extended time depressed, usually months, followed by periods of time when they are in an elevated, euphoric, and energized state referred to as mania. Most often, patients cycle from one type of mood to the other, often interspersed with periods of normal moods, but occasionally with interims of mixed states, showing features of both depressive and elevated mood states simultaneously or in rapid succession.

The elevated moods form a continuum from increased energy, euphoria, irritability, and decreased sleep called hypomania to a more extreme condition complicated by hallucinations, delusions, disordered thinking, and disorganized and sometimes violently agitated behavior, which is called mania. Hypomania is characterized by euphoria, an inflated self-attitude, and an elevated vital sense. Patients feel elated, energized, and as if they are functioning better than usual. Their thoughts are sped up and horizons are expanded, such that the patient feels many brilliant ideas and opportunities are coming to him or her in rapid succession. Often, a noticeable increase takes place in the amount and speed of speech; interrupting these patients to obtain necessary information is difficult to accomplish. Because their energy is so high, patients feel a decreased need for sleep, and occasionally do not sleep at all.

When these symptoms impair judgment and function is lost, the patient is seen to be along the spectrum in the syndrome of mania. Manic patients not only have pressured speech but also often demonstrate a disorder of thought in which ideas come so fast that it is impossible to see the connections between them, a so-called flight of ideas. The expansive self-attitude may take on proportions outside the realm of reality, known as grandiose delusions. Paranoid delusional thoughts and/or hallucinatory experiences also occur in some patients.

Bipolar disorder has a genetic component, since it runs in families. In addition, in some families an effect called *anticipation* may occur in which the disease occurs at earlier ages in each subsequent generation.[35,36] In general, the onset of the illness takes place in late adolescence and early adulthood. Episodes of bipolar illness likely follow a kindling model, with earlier episodes requiring more psychosocial stressors for initiation, whereas later episodes require less provocation.[37]

In contrast to the familial bipolar disorder found in the general population, another type of mania appears to be specifically associated with late-stage HIV infection (CD4 count less than 200 per mm^3), and it occurs in cognitive impairment or dementia.[38] This syndrome is called AIDS mania and probably represents a related but different condition, as the patients show a lack of previous episodes or family history.[39] Clinically, patients with AIDS mania may be difficult to distinguish from those with delirium, as the sleep-wake cycle is often disturbed and patients show a good deal of confusion and cognitive impairment. For this reason, the work-up begins with a careful evaluation of the causes of delirium. Patients with AIDS mania may differ clinically from those with familial bipolar disorder, as the predominant mood tends to be irritability rather than elation or euphoria.

Depressive episodes are considerably more complicated to treat in patients with bipolar disorder than in those with major depression. It is useful to have a psychiatric consultation before treatment starts. The mainstay of treatment is still aggressive antidepressant therapy, but other drugs, particularly mood stabilizers such as lithium and valproic acid, are important in these patients as well.

The prevalence of bipolar disorder in HIV-infected populations has been estimated at 8 percent, which is more than 10 times the 6-month prevalence in the general population. This prevalence, however, includes both familial-type bipolar disorder and AIDS mania.[40] Manic episodes may lead patients to high-risk behaviors because of impulsiveness and excitability,[41] thus increasing the prevalence of the familial type of disorder in the HIV population. Both familial-type and AIDS mania-type manic syndromes put patients at risk for nonadherence to treatment, thus increasing the illness burden of the patient and potentially leading to further impairments of judgment that may cause high-risk behavior to continue, thus propagating the epidemic.

The treatment of mania in early-stage HIV infection is not substantially different from the standard treatment of bipolar disorder. Antipsychotic medications are particularly useful in stopping a manic episode, while mood-stabilizing agents (such as lithium salts) and anticonvulsant agents (such as valproic acid, carbamazepine, and possibly lamotrigine, gabapentin, and topiramate) may relieve manic episodes also, but they are often used to try to prevent further episodes of illness. Mood stabilizers can be safely prescribed for HIV-infected patients, but some potential interactions with antiretrovirals should be considered. These potential interactions are shown in Table 3.1.

As HIV illness progresses, mood stabilizers become more complicated, as many of these agents have significant side effects and may even cause delirium in patients with dementia. Therefore, in late-stage AIDS, and particularly in AIDS mania, antipsychotics play a key role in both the treatment of acute episodes and the prevention of recurrence. Although several years ago haloperidol and fluphenizine were the drugs of choice for their relatively "clean" profiles, the newer, atypical antipsychotics, such as risperidone, olanzapine, quetiapine, ziprasidone, and aripiprazole have become staples of treatment. The advantage of these atypical agents over older antipsychotics is mostly in the lower incidence of tardive dyskinesia, the late onset of involuntary movements, usually of the face and mouth but occasionally of hands, feet, and limbs. Specifically, however, olanzapine is sedating and promotes weight gain; thus, it is useful for emaciated patients who are not sleeping well. Quetiapine can be sedating but causes less

Table 3.1. Drugs used for mania

Medication	Starting dose	Serum level	Advantages/Side Effects	Interaction with HAART
Lithium	150 to 300 mg BID	0.8 to 1.2 meq/L	Thirst, nausea, polyuria, weight gain, acne, tremor, diabetes insipidus, hypothyroidism	None known
Sodium Divalproex	125 to 250 mg BID	50 to 150 ng/dL	Sedation, weight gain, dose-related tremor, hair loss, transaminase elevation, pancreatitis (rare)	Abacavir may increase valproate levels; ritonavir decreases valproate levels. *Valproate significantly increases zidovudine levels,*[1,2] *case report of hepatotoxicity because of combination of valproate, ritonavir, and nevirapine.*[3]
Carbamazepine	100 to 200 mg BID	8 to 12 ng/dL	Sedation, weight gain, dose-related tremor, agranulocytosis (rare)	Lamivudine and ritonavir may significantly increase carbamazepine levels; amprenavir, delavirdine, efavirenz, indinavir, nevirapine, and saquinavir may increase carbamazepine levels; carbamazepine may decrease amprenavir, delavirdine, efavirenz, *indinavir,*[4] lopinavir, nelfinavir, nevirapine, ritonavir, and saquinavir levels.
Gabapentin	100 to 300 mg TID	Unclear	Sedation, headache, weight gain	Gabapentin absorption is decreased when coadministered with Videx tablets because of antacid buffers.
Lamotrigine	25 to 50 mg BID	Unclear	Rash, weight gain, Stevens-Johnson syndrome	Ritonavir may decrease lamotrigine levels; abacavir may increase lamotrigine levels.

Source: Adapted with permission from Bartlett JG, and Gallant JE *2001–2002 Medical Management of HIV Infection.* Johns Hopkins University, Division of Infectious Diseases, 2001.

Note: Information on drug interactions that is not specifically referenced is based on knowledge of drug metabolism taken from package inserts and Internet sources and is of unclear clinical significance in most cases. Prescribers should read all package insert information before prescribing any medication.

[1]Lertora JJ, Rege AB, Greenspan DL, Akula S, George WJ, Hyslop NE Jr., and Agrawal KC 1994. Pharmacokinetic interaction between zidovudine and valproic acid in patients infected with human immunodeficiency virus. *Clinical Pharmacology and Therapeutics* 56:272–78.

[2]Akula SK, Rege AB, Dreisbach AW, Dejace PM, and Lertora JJ. 1997. Valproic acid increases cerebrospinal fluid zidovudine levels in a patient with AIDS. *American Journal of Medical Science* 313:244–46.

[3]Cozza KL, Swanton EJ, and Humphreys CW. 2000. Hepatotoxicity with combination of valproic acid, ritonavir and nevirapine: A case report. *Psychosomatics* 41:452–53.

[4]Hugen PW, Burger DM, Brinkman K, ter Hofstede HJ, Schuurman R, Koopmans PP, and Hekster YA. 2000. Carbemazepine-indiavir interaction causes antiretroviral therapy failure. *Annals of Pharmacotherapy* 34:465–70.

weight gain and might have a specific advantage in patients who need to sleep but not gain weight. Ziprasidone can be mildly activating in some patients and therefore may be of advantage in irritable AIDS mania patients demonstrating a lot of fatigue. For most cases of bipolar disorder and AIDS mania, however, expert psychiatric consultation is required.

Schizophrenia

Schizophrenia is a chronic disorder that may be described as a disease of executive function, the ability to plan and carry out complex tasks using adaptability to internal and environmental cues. It occurs in about 1 percent of people worldwide. The essential deficit is the inability to plan and carry out complex tasks that require the ability to respond appropriately to certain variables, such as understanding and using social cues and organizing goal-directed behavior. The disease is characterized by episodes of psychosis in which patients develop hallucinations (usually auditory), delusions (often paranoid and bizarre), and disordered thinking. Over time, most patients develop apathy, withdraw from social functioning, and become increasingly disconnected in social interactions. The disease onset usually occurs in the teens to twenties for men and in the twenties to thirties for women. Patients are often described as having been odd and withdrawn before the development of psychotic symptoms. The condition is a lifelong illness and is progressively disabling in most patients. Although severe forms of bipolar disorder can be equally disabling, the term "chronically mentally ill" usually is used to describe populations made up in large part of patients with schizophrenia.

Chronic Mental Illness and Sexual High-Risk Behavior

Chronically mentally ill patients have high rates of risky sexual behavior. Several studies have been done on patients with schizophrenia and chronic mental illness to assess their risk factors for HIV. These studies found high rates of multiple partners, alcohol and drug use during sex, trading sex for money, drugs, or a place to stay, sex with high-risk or known infected partners, and unprotected sex.[42-45] It is therefore not surprising that the prevalence of HIV in chronically mentally ill patients has been reported to be between 4 and 20 percent.[46-50]

Many reasons for the increased high-risk behaviors in this group have been established. Several studies have found that patients with schizophrenia had significantly less knowledge about AIDS and HIV infection than control subjects or patients with other psychiatric disorders.[51-53] However, one of these studies found that AIDS knowledge did not correlate with behavior changes for patients with a psychiatric disorder, in contrast to control subjects. Changes in the sexual behavior of schizophrenic patients correlated with perceptions of cognitive control, a belief that one can reduce one's risk of AIDS by changing one's behavior, and a belief in the future development of advances in medical treatment for AIDS.[54] Additionally, it has been suggested that AIDS knowledge is not the only factor in lowering high-risk behavior, as some samples have found higher rates of risk behaviors despite a greater understanding of AIDS risk.[55]

It has been proposed that schizophrenic patients have high rates of homosexual behavior,[56-59] but other studies have found that the incidence of this among patients with other psychiatric illnesses was higher than among schizophrenics.[60] The commonly accepted idea that patients with bipolar disorder are at an increased risk for HIV because of hypersexuality during manic episodes is variably supported by data.[61-63] Our literature search revealed only one multiple-patient study that definitively correlated a diagnosis or symptomatology with high-risk behavior.

In a survey of 178 patients from multiple settings, McKinnon et al. found that the chances of trading sex were increased 3.5 times for patients with schizophrenia. Using the Positive and Negative Symptom Scale, the presence of more positive symptoms (delusions, unusual thought content, grandiosity, suspiciousness/persecution) increased the relative risk of multiple partners by nearly threefold. More excitement symptoms (excitement, poor impulse control, hostility, tension) increased the relative risk of being sexually active by twofold and trading sex by more than fivefold, although a diagnosis of bipolar disorder did not correlate with sexual activity. Greater AIDS knowledge increased the relative risk of being sexually active by threefold. Notably, condoms were used by less than half of the sample population, and this fact did not correlate with any diagnosis, symptomatology, or AIDS knowledge.[41] We agree with all the authors that if definite psychosis-related reasons for risk behaviors are found, treatment of the psychosis is paramount to success in reducing high-risk behaviors.

In addition to deficits in HIV knowledge and increases in sexual behavior in general, several authors have described issues related to high-risk behavior. These studies have variably shown sociocultural issues play a role in condom use.[64,65] Although such issues may affect condom use in any population, the chronically mentally ill appear to have higher rates of risk behaviors such as trading sex for money or other goods. In addition, chronically mentally ill patients appear to have a greater risk of contracting HIV if they meet sex partners at psychiatric clinics.[66] This ties in well with the commonly accepted notion that chronically mentally ill patients have severe disruptions in their social functioning and may select sex partners from the pool of psychiatric patients because of availability and acceptance of their symptoms.

Intervention sessions directed at teaching patients about safer sex practices and improved sexual hygiene have been described.[67,68] Some studies have shown that such interventions have resulted in increased knowledge or decreased risk behaviors for chronically mentally ill patients[69,70] with no detriment to the patients because of the emotionally charged nature of the sessions.[71] All authors agree that programs to educate chronically mentally ill patients should be tailored to their specific needs. This means that the specific behaviors reported previously, such as coerced sex, multiple partners, partner choice, trading sex, drug use during sex, and so on, need to be addressed in the sessions. Also, providers must be prepared for the patients' learning impediments, such as thought disorders and delusional concepts, which, as stated above, need to be optimally treated by appropriate medical interventions. Condoms should be distributed, and their proper application demonstrated and practiced using anatomical models.

Chronic Mental Illness and Intravenous Drug Use

Numerous studies have shown that patients with schizophrenia and other chronic mental illnesses have high rates of substance abuse.[72-83] Various explanations have been proposed for the use of substances by psychiatric patients. First among these is the idea that mentally ill patients "self-medicate" with substances, attempting to alleviate symptoms or side effects of medicines.[84] The next most popular is the notion that chronically ill patients have disruptions of social functioning and use substances as a means of connecting with others.[85] These explanations help clinicians to treat dually diagnosed patients, but the fact remains that patients with major mental illnesses use substances frequently and therefore may be at a higher risk for HIV.

Substance abuse as a vector for HIV will be discussed in Chapter 5. However, the increased risk for HIV associated with addictions may also have secondary ramifications in patients with chronic mental illness. Studies have shown that concurrent substance abuse/dependence is associated with a more severe course of illness[86,87] and poor medication compliance.[78] Thus, substance abuse, by worsening psychiatric disorders, may cause more symptoms or worsen one's coping ability and lead to increased high-risk behavior.

Chronic Mental Illness and Medical Care

Chronically mentally ill persons have a poor appreciation of health care issues, and facilities providing treatment for psychiatric disorders are generally inadequate in their screening for HIV. Such patients may receive limited medical attention in general and therefore are at risk for sequelae of undiagnosed disorders, such as neurosyphilis and chronic pelvic inflammatory disease. Women with chronic psychiatric illnesses are less likely to receive prenatal care during pregnancy[65] and thus are more likely to spread any infection to their offspring. We emphasize that psychiatric providers should be vigilant for medical illnesses, even using a standard medical review questionnaire for the periodic assessment of a patient's medical status. In addition, we urge medical providers in clinics to spend extra care in examining the chronically mentally ill, because often their illnesses, or the stigma attached to them, prevent open lines of communication.

Treatment of Schizophrenia in HIV-Infected Patients

No current significant difference exists between the pharmacologic treatment of schizophrenia in an HIV-infected individual and the treatment of a noninfected person. Occasionally, issues arise because of delusions the schizophrenic patient has concerning the HIV infection itself. The most common of these is the belief that he or she does not have an HIV infection and that "all of this is a hoax," created to monitor the patient's activity or some other paranoid explanation. Treatment principles for patients with schizophrenia apply universally. They include medications for the control of hallucinations, delusions, thought disorders, and negative symptoms, as well as psychosocial rehabilitation for reintegration into the community. Reality testing should be supported at all times, and the confrontation of delusional thoughts should be gentle and appropriately timed.

Panic Disorder

For the most part, panic disorder and panic attacks are beyond the scope of this book. We have included this brief segment because the first patient we cared for was referred for panic attacks in 1988 (to GT), and this diagnosis often results as a medical rather than a psychiatric complaint.

Panic attacks are paroxysmal episodes of severe anxiety, overwhelming dread, a sense that something is terribly wrong, and panic. They are usually accompanied by a pounding heart, chest tightness (or even pain), difficulty breathing (or shortness of breath), dizziness, and sometimes other autonomic symptoms such as a sudden need to urinate, defecate, and even uncontrolled diarrhea. Patients often dread returning to a place where they have had such an attack and can rapidly become housebound because of the attacks, a condition called agoraphobia. They may come to the emergency department, convinced they are having a heart attack or dying. The attacks are usually short lived, lasting minutes, but the sense of overwhelming dysphoria and distress often persists for several hours. Many patients can recall the location, time of day, and date of their first attack many years later and can describe it in detail.

Untreated, patients have significant morbidity in terms of social isolation, loss of access to health care, and substance abuse. Attacks can be aborted by sedative hypnotic agents (including alcohol) but will persist without definitive treatment. Behavioral interventions such as graded relaxation and self-hypnosis are as effective as medication treatment for these attacks, if somewhat less convenient. The use of antidepressants for treatment (and sometimes the use of benzodiazepines to abort attacks acutely) are the pharmacologic interventions most often used. Not all antidepressants are equally effective, and expert consultation is recommended for treating this condition.

Obsessive-Compulsive Disorder

Obsessive-compulsive disorder (OCD) is an intriguing psychiatric syndrome that has been relatively uncommon in our clinical experience and has an unknown prevalence in HIV clinics. It is included in this discussion because many of the patients who have it never describe it to their doctor, and we have incidentally discovered the symptoms in several patients who initially failed to report them despite earlier psychiatric treatments.

OCD can be a significant barrier to adherence in HIV as patients may endlessly debate starting and continuing treatment. It can also be a source of much confusion for a subset of patients with sexual obsessions and rituals who may present with odd requests, concerns, and behaviors that may baffle clinicians. Also worthy of note is the fact that some patients with this disorder may become nearly delusionally convinced that they have AIDS or HIV when they do not, and may not even have any risk factors. The term FRAIDS (afraid of AIDS) has occasionally been applied to these patients. They may appear repeatedly for testing, attempting to be reassured that you are certain they do not have HIV.

The morbidity of OCD is impressive, but patients may have trouble accepting the diagnosis. It is a condition for which patients rarely seek help. Although they are often reluctant to accept it, referral for expert psychiatric treatment is important, and patients who receive treatment have improvements in symptoms and quality of life.

Case: Psychosis

C was originally seen by our group in 1992, when he was 31 years old. He was referred by an experienced and competent clinician who had become extremely upset when she discovered he was injecting drugs into the granulation tissues at the edges of the abscesses on his leg. These abscesses were the result of unclean injections, but the patient may have deliberately produced them. After this discovery, she decided he needed to be seen by the psychiatry service.

C's family history includes a brother who committed suicide, a second brother with schizophrenia, and several other siblings with substance use disorders. C grew up in a physically abusive and violent household with many disruptive parental changes. In the seventh grade, he was held back several times related to alcohol abuse and behavior problems. His first inpatient detoxification was at age 17. In his midteen years, he began to have auditory hallucinations and display odd as well as violent behavior. He began using heroin and cocaine at the age of 12, and it was unclear at the time whether the onset of his mental illness was related to his substance use or a separate condition. As a teenager, he received a diagnosis of schizophrenia and was found to have HIV in 1985. He had been treated for exposure to tuberculosis, had multiple physical wounds, including several stab wounds, and spent extended periods in jail and prison related to drugs and violent behavior.

C had no consistent employment and was receiving SSI disability each month. He lived with a woman he referred to as his wife, although he had never been formally married and he had frequent violent altercations with her. She was also a daily intravenous heroin and cocaine user. She had worked as a prostitute when her funds were short, and on several occasions C had discovered her in his apartment with a customer, usually resulting in violence. In at least one of these altercations, she and C traded stab wounds with knives, and on one occasion she tied him up while she had sex with one of her clients, forcing him to watch, and then afterward tortured him with a knife, to the degree that he required hospitalization for surgical treatment.

C also has a life-long history of psychiatric disturbance. He had violent altercations in elementary school and junior high before leaving school. He had been hospitalized at both acute and long-term state facilities, as well as most of the psychiatric units in the city since his teens. His admitting diagnosis was always schizophrenia, and his admissions always were related to ongoing auditory hallucinations and paranoia.

At the time of his referral, C was injecting heroin and cocaine into the granulation tissues surrounding the ulcers on his leg. He said he could no longer access the veins in his body, although occasionally he would pay a "doctor," one of the people in the drug community who was capable of accessing difficult-to-hit veins, to inject his drugs for him. When he could not arrange this, he would "shoot into sores" so that he could get a better high than simple skin popping. He was living with his girlfriend, who had frequently asked him for money, but who also supplied him with money and drugs on occasion.

When he arrived for his evaluation, C was emaciated and filthy. His clothes were literally rotting off his body, and he was extremely suspicious and anxious. He admitted believing that doctors were part of a plot against him, that he was the subject of experiments by doctors, and that somehow his cocaine and heroin were being removed from syringes and being wasted. He said that sometimes he would draw up his drugs in the syringe, then look away, and when he looked back the drugs would be gone. It was something he could not explain but knew was the work of others intending him harm. He admitted to auditory hallucinations talking about and to him, sometimes telling him to kill himself, often commenting on his clothing and his behavior, and sometimes suggesting that he do violence to others. He admitted that he occasionally assaulted people, believing they had stolen his drugs or he had heard them think a bad thought about him. His cognitive examination revealed very limited intellectual functioning and difficulty with math, verbal manipulations, and abstractions. The initial diagnosis was schizophrenia and mild cognitive impairment.

Although we have an extremely strict personal policy never to give money or goods to patients, at the first interaction we took C downstairs in front of the hospital and bought him a hot dog from one of the street vendors. C returned the following week after treatment with fluphenazine, and we purchased a hot dog for him a second time. Over the next several years, C was intermittently involved in treatment with us.

C responded to the antipsychotic treatment with fluphenazine and was additionally treated with amitriptyline to help his low mood and his sleep. Receiving medications (and hot dogs) was predicated on a clean toxicology screen and abstinence from drugs. On several occasions, C remained drug-free for periods of time but eventually relapsed each time. He was admitted several times to the hospital, but often left as his paranoia escalated and he became convinced that doctors in the hospital were experimenting on him. After several years, he accepted aggressive treatment with nortriptyline and fluphenazine, and this resulted in complete resolution of his auditory hallucinations and delusions. He became confident, pleasant, and warm. This was quite a surprising transition to his treatment team. He remained cognitively limited.

C was also persuaded to enroll in a methadone program. When ill, he would insist that the nurses were stealing his methadone and he would become threatening, but the methadone counselor and program director stood by him and kept him in the program.

For the next several years, C exhibited a decreased level of paranoia and experienced a gradual improvement in mood. He mostly recovered from his drug-use disorder, although negative interactions with his wife usually resulted in relapses of several weeks at a time. On several occasions she returned home, seduced him sexually, and began bringing drugs and the drug-related activities of prostitution into his apartment. She would also openly express her contempt for C and mistreat him. During these times, he would become demoralized and begin using drugs with her again. These episodes became less frequent and shorter in duration but continued to occur for several years. Ultimately, he was able to break from her entirely, and he has remained sober since that time.

In one striking episode, C had been doing well for approximately four months when he began to become paranoid despite a continued abstinence from drugs. He was admitted to the hospital and over the next several days his mood fell precipitously despite increases in his medication. On the sixth or seventh hospital day, he underwent an abrupt transition in which he became so paranoid as to frighten the staff and his physicians. He called for Dr. Treisman and told him everything the various staff members had done to him, and that he was afraid that if he stayed in the hospital he would eventually injure one of the doctors. He was allowed to leave against medical advice, only to return to the clinic approximately one week later greatly improved. He remained convinced for the next several months that his delusional ideas about what had happened in the hospital were true, and then abruptly all those delusional ideas melted away.

Unfortunately, after several years of taking nortriptyline, C developed acute urinary retention that resolved when his nortriptyline was stopped. He had several trials of selective serotonin reuptake inhibitor (SSRI) antidepressants with no improvement and was finally treated with nefazodone with trazodone for sleep. On this regimen he had another dramatic improvement and returned to his best level of functioning. On several occasions, he required dosage increases and ultimately ended up on a total dose of 1,200 mg of nefazodone per day (twice the highest recommended dose and partly because of a patient error in how he was taking his medication) with continued improved functioning. He eventually developed urinary retention on nefazodone, however, and is now awaiting prostate surgery while doing well on quetiapine, venlafaxine, and trazodone.

C has gained weight, his demeanor has improved over the years, and he is now an affable and healthy-looking man. On rare occasions his paranoia returns and at those times he can be quite frightening and agitated. Although he continues to have episodes of depression, he has not had auditory hallucinations in the last eight years. He has had several brief lapses of drug use, but he continues to come to the clinic once a month for medication and for occasional therapy.

Discussion

This case illustrates the complexity of both the diagnosis and treatment in an HIV clinic. It is one of many "hopeless" cases we have faced together. Although we often do not succeed in cases like this one, we have learned that we can be surprised by the outcome of a case if we simply do our best. It is often hard to say what the key to success is for a particular patient. In the following discussion, we give our thoughts on what we did correctly and why, but as C himself said once, "Maybe it was those hot dogs."

The issue of diagnosis in this case was particularly difficult. C has a major mental illness that produces intense paranoia and bizarre hallucinations and delusions. He is also socially withdrawn and dilapidated. These are consistent with his historical diagnosis of schizophrenia, but all of these symptoms began in the context of intense substance abuse. He has been free of these symptoms during antidepressant therapy without antipsychotic drugs for several years, but without nortriptyline he needs an antipsychotic to stay well. His odd and somewhat flat emotional tone improved off drugs and is absent now that he is well.

His diagnosis is complicated by his cognitive limitations, which place his IQ in the borderline range of intellectual functioning. It is unclear whether he has schizophrenia and major depression or just extremely severe major depression. Ultimately, we treated C as if he had both conditions, as well as severe cognitive impairment. This meant that all our efforts had to be explained carefully and repeatedly. It also meant that we had to be patient after episodes of paranoia, as C had little understanding of how severely his illness colored his experiences.

To some extent, this demonstrates the bias of physicians and their nihilism about certain conditions. We seem to feel that if he was this well with treatment, his condition could not have been schizophrenia. Years ago, a patient had a miraculous recovery from an adenocarcinoma with chemotherapy, and his resident doctor became convinced that the patient had not really had cancer. The doctor had a pathologist recheck the slides and, when the diagnosis was confirmed, decided that the specimens must have been mixed up. The idea of a miracle never entered his mind.

C clearly had a severe substance use disorder and was detoxified on repeated occasions. He initially would not consider a methadone program because the requirement of group attendance was daunting, but in the end this was very helpful to him. His cocaine abuse eventually declined as we required him to submit negative toxicology screens in order to receive methadone and treatment.

His coping skills and relationships needed intensive work in psychotherapy. This required that he be well enough to stay with a therapist for a few months without becoming paranoid, since initially his suspiciousness and hostility would be directed at the person working with him the most, such as his counselor at the methadone program, his therapist at our program, his nurse on the inpatient unit, or his doctor. He ultimately had to be convinced that his relationships needed to change and that he had to stop his sexual connections with drug-using women. He would be approached frequently for money by women needing drugs, begin relationships with them, and end up using drugs with them.

Finally, it was discovered that C expected his health care providers to ultimately abandon him. Because of changing insurance, medical care problems, and corporate health care ownership, it is difficult for even the highest-functioning patients to maintain a relationship with a health care provider. Without his clinician's commitment to him, he never would have received the care he needed. He recognized this and said that the single most important thing for his recovery was that, "You didn't never leave me. Most people don't never get someone like that." He requested the opportunity to be in this book, and his remarks are included below.

We would add that he is our most frightening patient. The transformation from the sweet, gentle, meek, and self-effacing person to the belligerent, paranoid, hostile, and physically threatening patient is terrifying to watch. He has on several occasions quit treatment, only to return contrite, apologetic, and confused about what happened. The fact that the staff have stayed with him, continue to treat him, and take the risk of caring for him is remarkable.

Patient's Commentary

"When I first came here, I was shooting up in abscesses, and I had two or three abscesses they had to bust right away. Then the infection got into my heart five different times. I almost had my legs cut off and my arms cut off because the infection went into them and then I almost lost my foot. I was so addicted to heroin and cocaine that I was shooting up water from the floor because I thought I had lost some of my coke. Then I had me shooting up toilet water; then I came in the hospital because I was drawing up toilet water, thinking I might have wasted some drugs into it. My pressure was worse, I was suicidal, and I wanted to hurt people. I was getting confused. I thought, 'Why things gotta be this way?'

"As I started to come and work with you, things got better, but then I would slack off and get sick again. I was scared when I was sick. I wasn't sure about nothing. Didn't know who did what or didn't do what, and [had] all kinds of thoughts about what people were doing to me. I couldn't eat or sleep, stayed up crying, and sat morning and night. I get myself into trouble and I get violent. It is the dark, the darkest time.

"Most people don't never get to see it when they get well. They stay sick and be sick all through their whole lives. I got well, off of drugs, got my life back. What helped me was you all stood by me, didn't give up on me, and now I feel pretty good most of the time."

Chapter Four
Personality in the HIV Clinic

with Heidi Hutton, Ph.D.

William Osler, perhaps the greatest physician of the twentieth century, said that it is more important to know what sort of person has a disease than to know what sort of disease a person has. He was speaking as an experienced clinician who knew that patients respond differently to various experiences. In short, it is possible to "know" a person, that is, to expect a characteristic type of response from him or her in a given circumstance. Although one cannot predict behavior with certainty in a specific instance, one can expect certain general patterns of behavior from a particular person. Thus, an understanding of how someone responds to circumstances, problems, and conflicts can lead clinicians to a more effective way of helping this person change his or her behavior.

We have found an understanding of the building blocks of personality extremely useful in the care of patients. We define personality as the emotional and behavioral characteristics or traits that constitute stable and predictable ways in which an individual relates to, perceives, and thinks about the environment and the self.[1-3] Among our patients, certain personality traits increase the likelihood of engaging in problematic behaviors such as potential HIV exposure, poor compliance with medication regimens, and difficulty working with health care providers.

Understanding personality traits when working with HIV-infected patients is useful for developing specific, effective risk-reduction strategies in order to achieve the best overall outcome. This chapter describes what we have found to be a coherent and useful approach to examining a patient's personality and its relationship to risky behavior, clinical interactions, and adherence to medication. Finally, we discuss effective core treatment strategies for managing patients with destructive personalities.

The Nature of Personality

Theories on personality began with the early classical scholars, such as Hippocrates, Plato, and Aristotle, and were followed by the contributions of numerous other theorists such as Aquinas, Hobbes, Nietzsche, Locke, and Machiavelli. Their incisive descriptions are still seen in contemporary observations of personality types. In the last half-century, psychiatry and psychology have developed useful approaches to the study of personality, but they have developed little consensus on how to define personality, what is a disordered personality, and what is actually wrong with a patient who has such a disorder.

Psychodynamic theorists of the early twentieth century used clinical observations to describe the nature of personality. Sigmund Freud, Carl Jung, Melanie Klein, Otto Kernberg, and Erich Fromm hypothesized that the fundamental determinants of personality are rooted in early childhood experiences and that such experiences are combined with unconscious biological drives to produce lifelong behavior patterns. Behavioral theorists of the middle twentieth century rejected the notions of an internal psychological drive or unconscious motivations and argued instead that behavior is determined by the environmental contingencies of reward and punishment.

Current personality theory begins with the work of Gordon Allport in the 1940s and 1950s. His trait theory, as well as the work of Raymond Cattell, Hans Eysenck, Robert Cloninger, Theodore Millon, and Paul Costa, focuses on defining and quantitatively measuring personality traits. These personality theories are based on the ideas that (1) there are core personality traits and (2) these traits vary in individuals along a continuum or dimension and occur in the population with a mathematically normal or graded distribution.

Height and intelligence are examples of traits that occur on a continuum. Individuals vary as to how much of a trait they possess, with most people having an average amount, whereas the rest of the population has less or more than the average. Fig. 4.1 represents a theoretical curve for any given trait, such as height. Most people can be considered average, with just as many people below average as above average.

The average also represents the best survival advantage in an average environment. Such traits provide the best chance of survival over generations and through a variety of changing environmental conditions. Short stature, for example, may make a person vulnerable in times when food is high on a tree branch and out of reach. However, short stature may be very advantageous under harsher environmental conditions when survival depends on using less food and water becomes scarce.

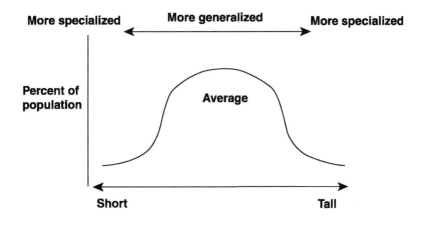

Fig. 4.1. Dimensional distribution of human traits: height

Smart people, such as those who originally developed IQ curves, do very well in environments that require abstraction, but they may be ill equipped to survive when one needs to think concretely about a problem. Digging enough potatoes to survive might require determination, perseverance, and resilience, but not necessarily brilliance. Those at the ends of the curve who represent the small populations of individuals with extreme endowments are extremely well adapted to certain special environments and tasks but poorly adapted to most others.

The study of personality is fundamentally about the function and adjustment of traits in an individual and his or her interaction with the environment. An excessive endowment of a particular trait or traits does not make one sick or disordered; it instead makes one well suited to a particular challenge in a certain kind of environment. This also makes one particularly poor at responding to another type of challenge, leading to vulnerability in circumstances where one is at a disadvantage. The greater the advantage a person has in one type of environment, the greater the disadvantage he or she will have in the opposite type of environment. A person can overcome his trait and thrive in environments where he or she is at a disadvantage, but the individual has to work harder than someone who naturally adapts to that environment.

Many of us see the traits themselves as neither good nor bad until subjected to a specific environmental set of stresses. When discussing the vulnerabilities of a particular trait, is it easy to lose sight of the assets that the trait confers, and for the demoralized patient struggling with that trait, it is easy for them to lose sight of their own assets as well. It is important to emphasize the neutral nature of the traits so that their assets can be appreciated along with their vulnerabilities.

Core Dimensions and Traits of Personality

In our discussion of personality, we will simplify several possible complex hypotheses to propose that personality is made up of two main components: temperament and character. Temperament is defined as the typical emotional responsiveness of a person—what types of things elicit emotional responses and to what degree, the intensity of the emotional responsiveness, and the salience of the emotional response to the person's likelihood of responding to the emotion. We will discuss the endowment of temperament in detail shortly. Character is a set of values, ethics, and morals that act as guidelines within which temperament can determine responses to stimulus. For example, a person with an extraverted style might be driven to take a risk based on the emotions the situation generates, but his or her character might reject the urge to act and the rationalization of acting because of a strong moral opposition. In this model it is important to understand that temperament is an innate endowment—it is not easily changed over the lifespan and is thus the nature part of personality development, but character is learned and makes up the nurture part.

Most personality theories depict individuals' temperament along dimensions of (1) *extraversion/introversion* and (2) *stability/instability*.[4-7] The dimension of extraversion/introversion refers to the individual's basic tendency to respond to stimuli with either excitation or inhibition. Individuals who are extraverted respond with excitement or activation and are (1) present oriented, (2) feeling directed, and (3) reward seeking (Table 4.1).[8-10] Their chief focus is their immediate and emotional experience. Feelings have primacy over thoughts, and the predominant motivation is immediate gratification or relief from discomfort. Extraverted individuals are sociable, crave excitement, take risks, and act impul-

Table 4.1. Distinctions between extraversion and introversion

Extraversion	Introversion
Present-time orientation	Past and future orientation
Feeling-directed	Thinking-directed
Reward-seeking	Consequence-avoidant

sively. They tend to be emotionally intense, charismatic, impulsive, risk taking, and optimistic.

Extraverts thrive in environments of change, risk, challenge, and creation. Successful extraverts can be found in the arts, sales and marketing, politics, and other jobs that require an ability to change rapidly, connect with others emotionally, and creatively respond to new challenges quickly. This is not to say that there are no extraverts who are accountants or doctors; there are just parts of those jobs that are more difficult for extraverts. The chief executive officer of an organization tends to be an extravert.

By contrast, introverted individuals respond to stimulation with inhibition and are (1) future and past oriented, (2) cognition directed, and (3) consequence avoidant. Logic and function predominate over feelings. Introverts are motivated by appraisal of a past experience and the avoidance of future consequences. They will refrain from a pleasurable activity if it might pose a threat in the future. Introverted individuals are quiet, dislike excitement, and distrust the impulse of the moment. They tend to be orderly, reliable, and rather pessimistic.

Introverts like orderly, stable, and clearly demarcated tasks and lives. Successful introverts tend to be found in law, accounting, medicine, and other jobs that involve careful and thoughtful styles. This is not to say that no introverts do stand-up comedy or are rock stars; there are simply harder parts of these jobs for an introvert. The chief financial officer of an organization tends to be an introvert.

In general, however, most of the population falls in the center area of the bell-shaped curve and has a more generalized endowment of temperament. This mixture of temperaments translates into an ability to adapt to the presenting circumstance with an appropriate temperamental style. A person with a modest amount of both introverted and extraverted traits (a middle-of-the-curve person) might find motivation in studying for a test so as not to fail (an introverted style), but after the test may enjoy going out dancing (an extraverted style).

At the extremes of the curves for these traits are those that are profoundly endowed with either introversion or extraversion (see Fig. 4.2). Here individuals are very well suited to only a very few occupations or pursuits, and find great difficulty in many of life's everyday tasks, since at the end of the curve, individuals have less ability to adapt to the opposite temperamental style when necessary. Extreme introverts may be paralyzed when faced with decisions if they do not have ample time to analyze for potential pitfalls, and extreme extraverts may act impulsively on feelings without weighing thoughts that could have prevented a bad outcome had they been taken into consideration.

A second personality dimension, stability/instability, defines the degree of emotional liability (see Fig. 4.3). The emotions of stable individuals are difficult to arouse, have a modest maximal response, and usually are aroused to a similar

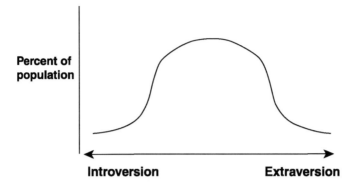

Fig. 4.2. Dimensional distribution of personality: introversion/extraversion

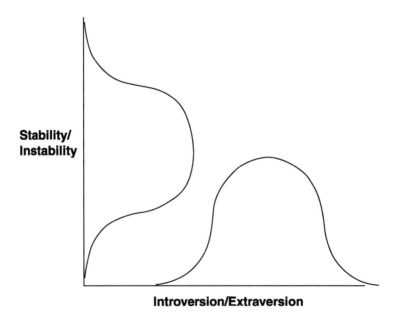

Fig. 4.3. Dimensional distribution of personality: stability/instability and introversion/extraversion

degree and in the same way by similar stimuli. They are aroused slowly and minimally and act emotionally infrequently. By contrast, the emotions of unstable
individuals are easy to arouse, have an intense maximal response, and are unpredictable in terms of the amount and type of emotional responses to stimuli.
Unstable individuals have intense, mercurial emotions and often act on them
impulsively.[7-9]

If these two personality dimensions are juxtaposed, four personality types
emerge (see Fig. 4.4). The inner circle shows Hippocrates's famous doctrine of
the four temperaments. The outer circle shows the results of numerous modern
experiments involving ratings and self-ratings of behavior patterns for large
groups of people.[9,11] The traits of these four personality types are distinctive, as
are their patterns of HIV risk or preventive behaviors.

Implications for HIV Risk Behavior

Of the four temperaments, unstable extraverts, or choleric types, are the most
prone to engage in HIV risk behavior. About 60 percent of the patients at the

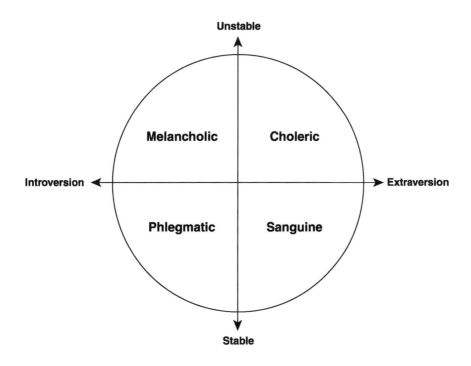

Fig. 4.4. The four-quadrant personality model

Johns Hopkins AIDS Psychiatry Service clinic present with this blend of extraversion and emotional instability. These individuals are preoccupied by and act on their feelings,[7,8,11] which are evanescent and changeable. Consequently, their actions tend to be unpredictable and inconsistent.

Perhaps most striking is the inconsistency between thought and behavior. Despite intellectual ability or knowledge of HIV, unstable extraverts can engage in behavior associated with extreme risks of HIV infection. Past experience and future consequences have little salience in decision making, and to individuals who are ruled by feeling, the present is paramount. Their overarching goal tends to be focused on the emotional needs of the present and is to achieve immediate pleasure or removal of pain, regardless of the circumstances.

Furthermore, as part of their emotional instability, they experience intense excursions in their mood. It is difficult for them to tolerate painful feelings, such as boredom, sadness, or unresolved cravings; they want to escape or avoid it as quickly and easily as possible. Thus, they are motivated to pursue pleasurable experiences, however risky, if they experience an improved mood or relief from discomfort.

Individuals who are present oriented, driven, reward seeking, and emotionally unstable are more likely to engage in behavior that places them at risk for HIV infection than stable introverts. Unstable extraverts are less likely to plan ahead and carry condoms and are more likely to have unprotected vaginal or anal sex. They are more fixed on the reward of sex and remarkably inattentive to the sexually transmitted disease they may acquire if they do not use a condom. Unstable extraverts are also less likely to accept the diminution of pleasure associated with the use of condoms or, once aroused, to interrupt the heat of the moment to use one. Similarly, unstable extraverts are more vulnerable to alcohol and drug abuse. They are drawn to alcohol and drugs as a quick route to pleasure. They are also likely to experiment with different kinds of drugs and to use greater quantities. In addition, unstable extraverts are likely to become injection drug users because the experience is more intense, and they are less likely to defer this intensity in the interest of safety.

The second most common personality type, representing about 25 percent of Johns Hopkins AIDS service patients, is the stable extravert. They too are present oriented and pleasure seeking; however, their emotions are not as intense, as easily provoked, or mercurial. Hence, they are not as strongly driven to achieve pleasure. Their emotional stability may generate a kind of indifference to HIV risk more than a drive to seek pleasure at any cost. Stable extraverts may be at risk because they are too optimistic or sanguine to believe that they will become HIV infected.

Introverted personalities are less common among Johns Hopkins AIDS Psychiatry Service patients. Their focus on the future, the avoidance of negative consequences, and a preference for cognition over feeling render them more likely to engage in protective and preventive behaviors than extraverts. HIV risks for introverts are largely determined by the dimension of emotional instability/stability or by the presence of other psychiatric disorders. About 14 percent of our patients present with a blend of introversion and instability, defined as the melancholic type. Unstable introverts are anxious, moody, and pessimistic. Typically, these patients engage in HIV risk behaviors not for pleasure, but for relief from pain that drugs or sex provides. They are concerned about the future and negative outcomes, but they believe they have little control over their fates. Thus, fatalism may interfere and reduce any consistency in their HIV-protective behaviors.

The remaining 1 percent of patients are stable introverts, or the phlegmatic type. These patients with their controlled, reliable, and even-tempered personalities are least likely to engage in risky or hedonistic behaviors. Typically, these individuals are HIV positive as a result of a blood transfusion or an occupational needle stick, but as we will describe in Chapter 5, they may engage in drug use when suffering from a major depression, for example, as the usual reward circuitry of the brain is dysfunctional and concomitant changes in outlook may lead to risky, albeit uncharacteristic, behavior.

Empirical investigation supports our clinical observations of the influence of extraversion and emotional instability on risky HIV-prone behavior. The Eysenck Personality Questionnaire (EPQ),[10] specifically developed to measure these traits, has high reliability and validity. High extraversion is associated with sexual promiscuity, a desire for sexual novelty, multiple sex partners,[12-14] and substance abuse.[16,17] Emotional instability is related to unsafe sex practices[6,14] as well as heroin addiction and other drug addictions.[16,18]

DSM-IV Personality Disorders in HIV-Infected Patients

The term *personality disorder* has been used to describe the problems that occur when personality traits exceed the average levels, are sufficiently extreme, and are maladaptive to cause subjective distress or functional impairments.[19,20]

We characterize our patients' temperaments along the dimensions of extraversion/introversion and emotional stability/instability, rather than in the discrete categories of behavior provided by Axis II of the *Diagnostic and Statistical Manual of Mental Disorders, Fourth Edition* (DSM-IV). We have found that personality traits do not represent discrete categories, but rather dimensions, and that patients have degrees of traits rather than personality disorders being an all-or-nothing phenomenon. It is easier, quicker, and more predictive of future responses for clinicians to determine where a patient falls along two dimensions than to evaluate each of the nine criteria to determine if a patient meets criteria for a diagnosis of borderline personality disorder. Additionally, the category-based personality disorders used by the DSM-IV suggest that patients with a personality disorder have a lack of something, rather than an excess of it. This is in part a residuum from the psychoanalytic ideas about personality disorders. In the psychoanalytic concept, character disorders resulted from a failure of a necessary completion of a developmental stage, thus rendering patients vulnerable to faulty emotional, moral, or social growth. The model we use emphasizes that each personality style has assets associated with it, but it also carries vulnerabilities.

One must consider the assets of extraversion for leadership, survival, innovation, performance, and empathy. Our patients have often survived years of drug addiction, and their personality structures, while making them vulnerable to addiction, enable them to survive in circumstances others would be unable to tolerate.

The dimensional model has three other advantages over the categorical model taken from the DSM-IV. First, by emphasizing the assets as well as the liabilities of personality traits, the dimensional model suggests both an explana-

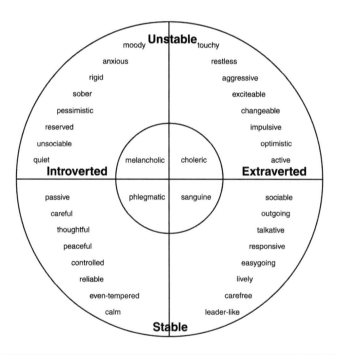

Fig. 4.5. Eysenck's personality circle

Source: Eysenck HJ. 1970. Principles and methods of personality description, classification and diagnosis. Chapter 3 in *Readings in Extraversion-Introversion, I. theoretical and Methodological Issues.* New York: Wiley-Interscience, p. 36.

tion of behavior and a set of interventions. Second, a diagnosis of an antisocial or borderline personality disorder has become a synonym for an untreatable condition and can be stigmatizing, particularly in a general medical clinic where care providers may have less experience managing such patients, once again a holdover from past ideas that character flaws could be rectified only with years of intensive sychoanalytic therapy, if at all. Finally, a classification system based on a continuum approach is a better predictor of risky HIV-prone behavior than DSM-IV Axis II categories.[21]

However, the DSM-IV method does have compelling uses despite these arguments. It provides a clear diagnostic set of criteria that are either met or not, thus enhancing the reliability of a diagnosis and helping in research studies. DSM-IV Axis II diagnoses are more often evaluated in research because the extremes of certain personality characteristics are easier to identify and measure, and they represent more disabling conditions. The method has good inter-rater reliability, and the diagnoses tend to be reliable and sustained over time. They predict behavior well in statistical models, and a good correlation exists between the dimensional model described previously and the categorical model of the DSM-IV if one translates them according to Fig. 4.4.

Approximately 10 percent of adults in the general, non-HIV-infected population have personality disorders,[22] whereas comparable prevalence rates of personality disorders among HIV-infected (19–36 percent) or at-risk (15–20 percent) adults are much higher.[23-25] The most common personality disorders among HIV-infected individuals are antisocial and borderline types.[26] In dimensional personality research, which specializes more than research into the overarching categories, antisocial individuals and those with borderline personality disorder score higher on extraversion scales and emotional instability scales.[7,9] Individuals with personality disorders have high rates of substance abuse,[27] a known risk factor for HIV infection.[28,29] Conversely, approximately half of drug abusers meet the criteria for a diagnosis of antisocial personality disorder.[30,31] Furthermore, individuals with a personality disorder, particularly an antisocial personality disorder, are more likely to inject drugs and share needles than those without an Axis II diagnosis.[32,33] This research supports our observations that personality affects HIV risks.

Implications for the Treatment of HIV-Infected Persons

Across a variety of diseases and patients, adherence to medication has been consistently estimated at 50 percent; that is, an average of half of the prescribed doses are taken by patients.[34] With HIV, adherence is especially challenging. HIV has all the components associated with low adherence: a long duration of treatment, preventative rather than curative treatments, asymptomatic periods, and frequent, complex medication dosing.[35-37] In HIV, estimates of adherence to zidovudine (AZT) vary widely, with patients taking from 26 to 94 percent of their prescribed doses.[38]

Our clinical experience suggests that nonadherence is more common among our extraverted or unstable patients. The same personality characteristics that place them at risk for HIV also reduce their ability to adhere to demanding drug regimens. Specifically, their present-time orientation, combined with reward seeking, makes it more difficult for these patients to tolerate uncomfortable side effects from drugs whose treatment produces benefits in the future but not in the present. It is also difficult for feeling-driven personalities to maintain consistent, well-ordered routines. Hence, following frequent, rigid dosing schedules can be problematic. Our unstable extraverted patients usually intend to follow the schedule, but their chaotic and mercurial emotions are likely to intervene and disrupt daily routines. For example, a patient may report that he felt very upset and nihilistic after a fight with a family member and thus missed several doses of his antiretroviral medicines. Missed doses of highly active antiretroviral therapy (HAART) can increase the chance of the HIV virus developing resistance. Recognizing factors that promote adherence to taking medication is important in improving a patient's overall outcomes.[39]

The psychiatric and medical treatment of patients with extraverted and/or emotionally unstable personalities is challenging. Many great physicians have commented on the types of patients they found to be difficult to treat. In the seventeenth century, the great physician Thomas Sydenham despaired of treating patients with difficult personality types. He summarized his experience with them by saying, "All is caprice. They love without measure those they will soon hate without reason. Now they will do this, now that; ever receding from their purpose."[40]

Personality disorders are confounding and demoralizing to medical providers. Clinicians are confused about what these conditions are, and an overwhelming mythology surrounds personality disorders. It is common to have a medical student or house staff member explain that these patients are untreatable or, having read some psychoanalytically focused literature on the subject, describe that the patients have a lacuna of the superego, a fragmented ego structure, or a psychotic core, all terms referring to severe character flaws or an inability to process information rationally. The impossibility of an effective treatment for patients with personality disorders is often taken with the certainty of physical laws of nature. Such patients are often baffling or frustrating for physicians and other medical providers because they engage in high-risk behaviors in spite of knowing the risks, or they fail to adhere to treatment regimens for HIV infection despite knowing the consequences. A patient may complain that a selective serotonin reuptake inhibitor (SSRI) gives him or her a mild headache while seemingly untroubled about injecting cocaine into his or her carotid artery. After 6 months of missed medical appointments, an unstable extravert may impulsively leave when the physician is 15 minutes late for their appointment. Such personality traits reflect relatively predictable lifelong modes of response; thus, direct efforts to change these traits are unlikely to be successful. It is possible, however, to modify the behavior that is an expression of the trait. By recognizing individual differences in risk-related personality characteristics, interventions can be better targeted and their effect maximized.

Introverted people tend to see the strength of their style in statements that emphasize a "look before you leap" approach or the fable of the grasshopper and the ant. Extraverts emphasize the strength of their style in phrases such as "he who hesitates is lost." Because health care providers are mostly introverted, they may have significant difficulty in seeing the positive aspects of extraversion.

Extraverts find their feelings important, are reward sensitive, and are focused on the present. They tend to act rather than not act. Clinicians, most of whom are introverts, are shaped by consequences and the future. They tend to emphasize function rather than feeling. With introverted patients, they are successful in changing behavior by focusing on risk, the possibility of dire consequences, and the future. When they warn an extraverted patient what will happen if she does not modify her behavior, they have little effect. Interaction with extraverts needs to focus on the desired rewards of behaviors, rather than the consequences of the behavior that should cease. In the domain of addressing medication adherence with an extravert, one can focus on positive features of taking medications, such as how many viral particles are destroyed if one takes all the medicine, the immune restoration that comes with successful treatment, and improvements likely to be seen with successful treatments. With introverts, as the treatment is successful, they improve with less clinical attention, whereas extraverts who are doing well may need more attention to maintain their commitment to treatment and continued progress, as, once the immediate rewards are over, the motivation to continue the behavior wanes.

Extraverts tend to arrive at a clinic already knowing what they want from the clinician. Rather than requesting medical treatment, they often arrive with forms they want filled out, demands for access to benefits (or the more politically correct but countertherapeutic term *entitlements*), and laundry lists of medications they need to take for unclear reasons, many of which are psychoactive medications of an unclear benefit. Some of these things can be used as the rewards the clinician can use to help motivate the patient to succeed in the treatment.

The initial step in treatment always involves an induction of the roles of clinician and patient. The diagnosis needs to be presented in a way that allows the patient to accept what is likely to be an uncomfortable treatment plan. Taking a careful history and performing a careful examination can help in designing an effective presentation of the diagnosis. This should include a description of what you think the problem is, how it is likely to be solved, and finally a strong message of encouragement accompanied by a clear list of treatment goals, rules, and expectations for both the doctor and patient. A useful technique for treating extraverted patients is to emphasize the fact that the patient has an extra endowment, an above-average amount of feelings, and that these feelings are directing his or her behavior. The provider can then cite examples from the patient's life when a bad outcome occurred and the patient was uncertain how he or she reached the bad outcome. An explanation that strong feelings led to the behavior that, in retrospect, was a bad choice, thus enables the patient to see how his or her endowment can be powerful, yet also sparks a desire to overcome the endowment when it acts as a liability. Describe the need to have a set of predetermined behavioral rules that can help lead to successful behaviors in emotionally charged situations, and discuss the likely types of rewards that will accumulate if the patient maintains the treatment course.

Experienced clinicians know that these patients require a great deal of attention for a successful treatment. To have any chance of success, the patients need to know what the clinician's goals are. They often wish to be made comfortable rather than better. Heath care is about health, not feelings, and the clear message has to be that "you will feel better when you get better." Efforts to feel better right now only lead to feeling worse later, but efforts to get better now will make the patient feel better later. We emphasize the following goals for treatment: function, longevity, and quality of life.

We have found that a cognitive behavioral approach is most effective in treating patients with extraverted and/or emotionally unstable personalities. Four principles inform our usual care:

- Focus on thoughts, not feelings. Unstable, extraverted personalities benefit from learning how they are predisposed to act in certain ways. Often, they recognize that they are highly emotional and are driven by their feelings. They may even be as baffled by their actions as the clinicians are. These patients fail to understand why, despite their intentions to stay clean, they later find themselves injecting drugs. The psychiatrist can identify the role that strong feelings play in their lives, so that these patients can begin the process of understanding their own self-destructive behavior. Patients can then focus on doing what is right or healthy, rather than what is immediately pleasurable. The task is to build consistency into their behavior.

- Use a behavioral contract. When angry or feeling overwhelmed, these patients sabotage their care. They act out their feelings toward the treatment staff, perhaps idealizing one staff member while hating another. They may have intense suicidal feelings and manipulate the staff with them, demanding unreasonable amounts of time and attention, calling staff members at home, and interrupting work with other patients. If they are addicted to medications or drugs, they often focus on getting medications and money to trade or buy drugs. They enlist the sympathy of staff members but often appeal to them to get resources that are destructive to the patient rather than constructive.

A behavioral contract can help curb these problems by outlining goals for treatment in behavioral terms. It should describe the roles of the patient and physician in clear terms. It should also specify what the staff will provide and what is expected of the patient. Although the patient and psychiatrist may develop the contract, the focus of the treatment is *not* on what patients want or are willing to do to get off of drugs, but rather on the established methods that will be used, such as drug treatment and Narcotics Anonymous or Alcoholics Anonymous. The importance of the behavioral contract lies in the creation of a stable plan that supersedes the emotional meanderings of these patients who present an ever-changing array of concerns and priorities. The task of the psychiatrist is to order the priorities with a patient and help him or her follow through on them, regardless of changing emotions. In short, behavioral contacts provide a consistent, cognitive focus to patients' bewildering emotional approach to life.

- Emphasize rewards. The behavioral contract should be presented to patients in terms of the rewards they will reap when they change their behavior. Positive outcomes, not adverse consequences, are salient to extraverts. For example, extraverts usually must be persuaded to wear condoms to avoid sexually transmitted diseases (STDs), and success has been achieved by eroticizing the use of condoms[41] or by the addition of novel techniques, such as erotic massage or the use of sex toys, to sexual repertoires.[42] Similarly, the rewards of abstaining from drugs or alcohol should be emphasized, as they would allow patients to have money to buy clothes, obtain a stable home, or help build positive relationships with children.

   In building adherence to antiretroviral therapies, the focus must be on the rewards of an increased CD4 count and a reduced viral load, rather than avoiding illness. Using the viral load as a strategy to build adherence can increase acceptance by all patients, but it is especially effective in reward-driven extraverts.

- Coordinate with medical care providers. As stated previously, medical care providers are often frustrated or discouraged by unstable, extraverted patients. It is particularly effective to develop a coordinated treatment plan, where a medical care provider and a psychiatrist work in tandem to develop behavioral contracts to reduce HIV risk behavior and build medication compliance. This can provide more consistency in care.

In practice, many patients rebel when the treatment contract conflicts with their immediate desire and wants. They initially see emotionally charged desires as needs and have no ability to tolerate frustration. In the context of a crisis, they will violate any agreement they have made and then explain that they had no choice. We explain to patients that this is unacceptable and point out that we continue to meet our portion of the treatment contract regardless of how we feel.

At this point, some patients will need to be discharged from care. Making a discharge a positive rather than an abandoning experience can be the most crucial step in treatment. We tell patients that we will gladly treat them if they honor the treatment plan we have made with them. We tell them they will be welcome to return to treatment if they agree to change their behavior. We understand their feelings, but if we tolerate actions driven by their feelings, it will lead to treatment failure, as it always has for them. Initial contracts are usually verbal agreements, but we often require a patient who has been discharged to write his or her own contract when he or she returns to try again. We tell patients that we will be glad to try again with them as often as they wish, but that we will not participate in treatment that will harm them, is futile, or is destructive to the clinic.

Conclusion

Behavioral change comes slowly and often requires a consistent effort over long periods of time. Patients may need to intermittently leave the clinic and go through several behavioral contracts before they can reliably maintain a relationship with the clinic. The keys to success are a firm set of expectations for improvements in behavior despite failed efforts and a willingness to focus on the treatment goals, not on the feelings generated by the patient. This also means that staff members need to be protected and supported in the often difficult interactions with patients. Good communication among staff members is needed to have clear ideas about what will be done in chaotic circumstances and patient crises.

Personality characteristics and disorders reflect relatively stable, lifelong propensities that are difficult to change. This does not mean, however, that HIV risk-reduction efforts are necessarily futile. Rather, by understanding personality characteristics and their role in risky behaviors and medication adherence, the psychiatrist can develop more effective, specific treatment strategies. Similarly, the HIV-positive patient who can identify the aspects of his or her personality that might interfere with intentions to practice safer behavior, and who knows strategies for dealing with these situations, is less likely to engage in high-risk behaviors. Finally, psychiatrists can provide valuable assistance to medical care providers in order to improve the health outcomes for these patients.

Case: Personality Disorder and Chronic Pain

D was a 37-year-old, single African American male when he was referred by his primary HIV provider to the AIDS Psychiatry Service for a "narcotic problem." At his first presentation, he arrived in an angry mood complaining of intractable chest pain. He had a long history of bullous lung disease and had chronic shortness of breath. He had been receiving oxycodone, sustained-release oxycodone (Oxycontin), hydrocodone, meperidine, propoxyphene, and methadone from a variety of providers in the clinic. He was angry about being "forced to see a shrink" and demanded refills of his narcotics or else he was not sure "what was going to happen."

D had a lifelong history of behavioral difficulties. Establishing an accurate family psychiatric history was nearly impossible, but he reported that his mother was an alcoholic. His father died at 32 of a stroke, leaving his mother and five children. His sister died of rheumatic heart disease at age 13 when D was 16. He quit school in the ninth grade after several years of fighting and other disciplinary problems to enter the job corps program, but he was expelled for fighting. Despite these difficulties, D was thought to be bright. He read and wrote well. He then entered the military but received a general discharge after two years because his girlfriend was pregnant and having medical problems. By his description, "After that, it was all downhill, with sex, drugs, and alcohol." He was subsequently married but divorced after nine years because of his ongoing infidelity. He had no children in that relationship but has two children from other relationships. He remains close with one child now.

At his evaluation, D was receiving public assistance for his lung disease. He had been living in a variety of housing situations, almost all of them alone. He had no hobbies. He had always worked as a cook, something in which he took great pride because he felt he was very good at it, but he was unable to work because of his lung disease. He had undergone a series of arrests starting in his teenage years, but denied ever serving time other than time awaiting trial, although records suggest he had been to prison.

D had been diagnosed with HIV in early 1997. He had received his diagnosis of bullous lung disease about 10 years earlier when he was suffering from a spontaneous pneumothorax. He had been told he had severe lung disease and would die within a year or two. He had developed a total of four spontaneous pneumothoraces requiring the placement of a chest tube and hospitalization. D reported chronic pain at the tube placement sites as well as diffuse chronic pain throughout his chest wall. He also had a history of multiple assaults with injuries. At the time of his evaluation D's CD4 count was 1680 cells per mm^3 with a viral load that was undetectable. His health care providers were convinced that most of his chronic chest pain was unrelated to his lung disease. They believed it to be exaggerated and related to old wounds and neuropathy.

D had a long history of alcohol and marijuana use dating back to his early teens. He also used cocaine several times a week, depending on the availability of drugs and funds, but denied injecting cocaine. He began using opiates in his teenage years, but his patterns of use and amounts were unclear. At the time of his evaluation, he was using only prescription opiates, but admitted he had used heroin in the past. He stated he was always able to get enough money to keep from having withdrawal symptoms. He also confessed he had recently met with increasing difficulties obtaining the money for adequate drug use. He drank alcohol but said it made him violent and he felt he "should just leave it alone." He had tried many other drugs but had no habits of using them. In addition, he smoked one to two packs of cigarettes per day.

His exam was significant for modest cachexia, a resting respiratory rate of 32 breaths a minute, and mild clubbing of his fingers, a sign of chronic hypoxia. He was irritable and contentious during the interview, frequently complaining of pain and wanting to stop the discussion. He had no thought disorder, his mood was described as "very up and down, but mostly down," and he stated he felt he was very ill. He denied any change in his attitude toward himself, but no longer had any hobbies or social activities in which he regularly engaged. His sleep was poor, he had a limited appetite, and he had been losing weight steadily for several years; at the time of his evalualtion he was 25 pounds lighter than when he was younger. He was cognitively intact with an above-average intellect and a better vocabulary than expected based on his education. Throughout the interview, he was extremely defensive about being sick and suggested he was not just another addict looking for drugs. Although he admitted to his addictions, he stated he needed opiates for his chest pain and that if his pain was under control he would no longer need other street drugs.

The team felt his diagnosis included antisocial personality disorder, probable major depression, opiate and cocaine dependence, and severe bullous lung disease. His lung disease caused chronic air hunger, a problem that causes severe anxiety or irritability in some patients. We were uncertain if he had a chronic pain disorder or was using his pain complaints to get opiates, because repeated work-ups had not demonstrated a reliable medical cause for his pain, but we included a diagnosis of chronic pain since it certainly merited attention.

We were quite confrontational with D during his first visit. We emphasized the question of whether he wanted to live or die, and that we wished to focus our treatment on life and improving his function, rather than simply providing comfort while he died slowly. We pointed out that he continued to smoke, that his drug-taking behavior was bad for his health, and that by demanding opiates he was distracting his medical care providers from thinking about his lung disease and HIV infection. We told him that if it were not for his drug addiction, his doctors would be very focused on his lung disease, his smoking, and his breathing.

We also discussed his psychiatric diagnoses. The conversation focused on addiction, major depression, and finally the differences between different personality types. We explained to him that people vary in the amount of traits they possess, such as intellectual prowess. Some people may be very smart and even gifted, whereas others struggle with limited intelligence to do what seems easy to those with a rich endowment of intellect. We then pointed out that the same is true of feelings, and that while one person may have limited feelings and is somewhat like a cold fish, another person might have lots of feelings and might even be called a "genius of emotions." We told him he was one of the people who had strong feelings, and that sometimes feelings as strong as these were hard to manage.

During the interview, we called his medical care providers and discussed all the options available for more effective treatment of his lung disease. D was quite clearly surprised when we discussed this, and it dramatically changed the atmosphere of the interaction. He was extremely interested in the possibility of improved breathing, and when we discussed the lack of clarity about his prognosis and that we were unsure how long he would live, he became quite interested in his pulmonary treatment options.

At the end of the interview, after we had begun several new bronchodilators, we discussed pain treatment. We spent time educating D about the acute exacerbation of pain he would commonly experience when he was in opiate withdrawal and that the management of chronic pain with opiates was different than the management of acute pain. We discussed a variety of nonopiate treatments for his chest pain in addition to opiates.

At the end of the first meeting, D was offered four different opiate choices for managing his pain: three Tylox (oxycodone plus acetominophen) pills a day to be taken at spaced intervals, sustained-release oxycodone (Oxycontin) to be taken twice a day, methadone to be taken twice a day, or a fentanyl (Duragesic) patch to be used every three days. He chose Tylox. We also offered him inpatient detoxification to address his addiction and clonidine to help with his opiate cravings. In addition, we recommended nortriptyline to treat his major depression and chronic pain. We pointed out that it was also likely to help him gain weight and sleep better and that we were able to monitor serum levels so we would know when he was at an optimal dose.

Initially, D was reluctant to accept treatment other than inhalers and opiates. He began to pick and choose which treatments he wanted, but we insisted the treatment was a package. He would not be required to take medication, but he would be required to give up the use of any medications or drugs other than those we prescribed. D would be required to come to the clinic for regular appointments where we would have ongoing discussions on his treatments and progress. At each visit he would be required to rate us as to how well we were doing in terms of his treatment, and he would take a urine test for toxicology screens. We told him we took his pain very seriously, but that he was unlikely to be pain free. D was told that with proper treatment he would no longer need to use street drugs and that we intended to make sure he got the best possible treatment. We added that if he thought we were not doing our very best, he should fire us and find doctors that he thought could do better. When we discussed the toxicology screens, D became angry and asked if we trusted him. We explained to him that it was important to document for everyone that he was not just a drug addict looking for narcotics, but we also added that, no, we did not trust him. We wanted to make sure his usual patterns of behavior did not sabotage his treatment, and that even though we knew he was sincere in his desire to get better, we wanted to prevent old habits driven by feelings of the moment from destroying his hard work and good intentions. He was able to accept this reluctantly, particularly when we pointed out how useful months of negative toxicology screens could be in court, "just in case any of your old life tries to reach out from the past and drag you back down." We also pointed out that he had no choice about this if he wanted prescription narcotics. This seemed satisfactory at the time of his first visit, and we did not insist on a toxicology screen at that time.

On the second visit, D admitted to supplementing his opiates with street heroin, but said he was already better and that the treatment was helping. He had not started the nortriptyline, but he had not used any cocaine for a week. We were very pleased that he was better and that he had resisted cocaine, but we could not give him opiates if he was using heroin, and we offered two choices: he could come in for a brief detoxification for three days or he could come to the clinic each day for a brief outpatient detoxification that would last one week. He elected outpatient detoxification and was given a one-day supply of clonidine, tylox, and diphenhydramine (Benadryl) and told to return to the clinic the next day. If he had any problems, he was directed to come to the emergency room and have them call us. The next day he returned and again received a one-day supply of medications. This time he was also given some dicyclomine (Bentyl) for nausea and cramps from mild withdrawal. On the third day he returned and had his first negative toxicology screen in his clinic history. He finished the outpatient detoxification and began to receive one-week supplies of medications the following week. He was continued on 0.3 mg of clonidine three times a day along with the oxycodone.

The third week he reported he lost his medications and asked for a resupply. This happened again the fourth week, and when confronted he admitted to taking all his medications at the first half of the week, thus running out and suffering withdrawal during the last two to three days. Again, we dealt with this by requiring daily clinic visits and offering inpatient treatment.

Over the next several months, D discontinued treatment on several occasions, only to reappear after a month or two and start over. Each time he was met with enthusiasm and encouragement, but strict rules. He also tested every rule, changing medications, getting medications from outside doctors, and running out of medications early because he had taken extra doses. Each time we complimented him on his honesty, but required daily visits until he was able to manage his medications correctly. He reported a slight improvement of his pain on nortriptyline and gabapentin (Neurontin) with no effect on his mood. He denied any improvement with carbamazepine, fluoxetine, paroxetine, valproic acid, and a variety of nonsteroidal anti-inflammatory drugs, but his sleep improved on a low dose of trazodone. He took each drug as a trial and eventually stayed on gabapentin and nortriptyline for about a year.

We also worked to optimize his breathing, which improved with the aggressive use of inhalers. D gained about 10 pounds, and his social functioning improved markedly. He was also able to obtain stable housing after about three months. During his treatment, he continued to have negative toxicology screens, but it seemed that he had reached a plateau without being able to improve in any other areas of his treatment.

D continued to smoke and developed an episode of bronchitis that responded well to nebulized bronchodilators. This was a turning point in his treatment. We suggested that we could get him a home nebulizer in exchange for him doing something for us. He initially offered to pay us a little cash but was surprised when we said that we meant he would have to quit smoking. We also pointed out that finding shortcuts was the way he saw the world, and he laughed while he recounted tales of bribing police officers, juvenile detention counselors, and other officials he had met. He eventually tapered off cigarettes and benefited from home nebulizer treatments.

After several years in treatment, D got into a fight with a former drug friend and was arrested. He was astonished when we offered to come to court on his behalf, but then said, "What's it going to cost me?" We made a deal that in exchange for a strongly worded letter to the court with accompanying documentation of negative toxicology screens, he would join a local church and do volunteer work. Although he hated this idea, he agreed to it. At church he met a woman who has now been his girlfriend for more than a year. She does not do drugs, drink, or tolerate much nonsense.

At his last clinic visit, D looked dramatically better than he did at the beginning of his treatment. He remains a somewhat isolated person who is still impaired by lung disease, but he is remarkably better now and is able to climb a flight of stairs. He occasionally requests a switch between sustained-release opiates to short-acting or back, but this occurs with far less frequency than in the past. Most notable is his intense pride in his improvement, his heightened self-esteem, and self-assurance. He graduated to a treatment plan in which he gives urine specimens for a toxicology screen and receives medications once a month. He is remarkably less guarded with health care providers and is caught smiling or even laughing once in a while.

Discussion

D presented with symptoms of problematic moods, but also clearly had intense feelings that ran his life. His medical care providers correctly made the diagnosis of antisocial personality disorder, but this had effectively prevented him from receiving anything other than palliative care for his lung disease. His demanding, hostile, and manipulative behavior had driven them to give him excessive opiates, which had not helped him get better. The team approach of enlisting all the health care providers to become involved in a plan consisting of firm limits was challenging regarding this patient. We placed a large note on his chart to call the psychiatry team before prescribing any narcotics for him, and his doctors needed constant encouragement to be involved in his care.

D is a reward-sensitive and punishment-insensitive person. His behavior had not been changed by violent beatings in childhood, juvenile detention as a teenager, or jail as an adult. He had also not been changed by the punishing losses of his personal life. Stab wounds, homelessness, lung disease, and HIV had little effect on his behavior. When he had failed several interventions with us and we were trying to think of what to do next, one member of our group joked that we could try shooting him in the leg because he had not been shot yet. Another person said that he probably had been shot but had neglected to tell us.

Keeping the team focused on firm rules but with positive reinforcement for D was difficult because it usually led to a struggle. He tested every rule and our standing response soon became, "We would be very sad if you fired us, because we think you should have a much better life and we could help you if you keep going." He remained a difficult and demanding person with lots of irritable outbursts and constant manipulation. Despite this, his health and life improved. He continued to have negative toxicology screens and developed a stable relationship with his girlfriend who seemed to provide real support for him.

The most interesting interactions D has at the clinic are with medical students, who get to hear the experience of treatment from his point of view. He tells them that when he first came the doctors were always fighting with him, giving him a hard time, and being belligerent. Over time, as he worked with the doctors, they understood him better and finally treated him with the right medications and in the right way, so he got better. "Now we get along well because they have changed the way they treat me."

He tells this story with a tongue-in-cheek delivery, knowing that his ability to change his behavior and maintain the change is what brought about the difference in his life. But his description is from the heart, as extraverts typically feel that they are the passive victims of circumstance, and cannot see how their own actions direct and cause the events or the setting in which the events occur. They make amazing statements, such as "I wouldn't have shot him if he hadn't made me mad" or "All of the sudden these three guys jumped me and beat me up." They do not see that they chose to carry a gun and to be in the company of violent and dangerous associates.

Ultimately, behavior is malleable while temperament remains fairly static. This patient sees the change in others but has difficulty seeing that he is responsible for the change. He will gladly take credit for the improvement, but still feels that somehow if he had just been treated differently and had different circumstances he would never have had difficulty in the first place. Although he can be persuaded to change his behavior, he never actually feels responsible for it.

In a sad addendum, after the writing of the manuscript for this book, D lost his temper with a social worker in the clinic and was expelled for the use of foul language and making threatening remarks. Despite this outburst, he asked to be included in this book anyway. He admitted that it was his own fault, and he is now working on a way to return to clinic. He feels that the most important messages for patients are "Don't let your feelings run your life" and "You've got to change what you do to change how you think."

Chapter Five
Substance Abuse and HIV

with Jeffery Hsu, M.D.

Alcoholism and substance use disorders are the focus of enormous energy and rhetoric by politicians and the medical bureaucracy. Despite public health efforts and some outstanding research on both the causes and treatment of addictions, the ability to translate research findings into meaningful programs has been complicated by politics and delayed by a lack of funding. The public view that these disorders are untreatable is incorrect. The lack of a coherent model that can incorporate the biological, psychological, sociological, genetic, and empathic roots of these disorders causes much confusion for those trying to understand these conditions. The costs of untreated drug and alcohol abuse are almost beyond calculation. They include the direct cost of the substances, which has now reached the billions, the cost of the crime related to paying for the drugs, and the cost of crime related to distribution of the substances. Additional factors include the costs of associated medical, social, educational, and occupational losses related to drug use, as well as the cost of the epidemic spread of infectious conditions like hepatitis C and HIV to non-drug-using sexual partners of addicted individuals.

In Baltimore City, with its estimated population of 650,000, there are between 25,000 and 35,000 daily injecting heroin users, each of whom spends an average of $40 per day on heroin. If one must sell about $400 a day of stolen property to get that $40, which is a reasonable estimate in Baltimore, and it costs about three times as much to replace a stolen article as to buy it (including the costs of insurance claims, repairs to doors and windows, and other costs), then the cost of the drugs alone in Baltimore is 365 multiplied by $1,200 a day, multiplied by 25,000 drug users. This astronomical cost is unthinkable in a poor city like Baltimore, which has terrible trouble supporting education, housing, and urban renewal. Books like *The Corner* and television shows like *Homicide* must actually downplay this reality to be believable. One inaccurate element of the portrayals of the addiction problem is the sense of hopelessness and untreatability they provoke. In years of working in an indigent AIDS clinic, we have seen many patients get off drugs, maintain sobriety, and develop independent lives. Our outcomes show that about one-third of our patients have attained and maintained sobriety.

Substance use disorders have always been closely linked to the human immunodeficiency virus (HIV) epidemic in North America. Unfortunately, despite great medical advances in the treatment of HIV infections in recent years, far less has been achieved in either preventing HIV infections among substance abusers or in treating substance use disorders in the HIV-infected population.

Injection drug use is obviously a primary means for contracting HIV. The proportion of injection drug users (IDUs) with HIV infections increased markedly from 17 percent during 1981–1987 to 33 percent during 1993–1995. In the city of Baltimore, approximately 75–80 percent of HIV positive individuals are IDUs.

Even among noninjection drug users, substance use plays a major, albeit more subtle, role in HIV transmission. Drug addiction and high-risk sexual behavior have been linked to HIV across a wide range of settings. For example, crack cocaine abusers are likely to engage in prostitution to obtain money for drugs. Alcohol intoxication can also lead to risky sexual behaviors by way of cognitive impairment and disinhibition. In a series of 250 patients presenting to our clinic for HIV care, gay men with no intravenous drug use still had a 75 percent rate of substance abuse, primarily using alcohol, cocaine, and benzodiazepines.

A Model for Understanding Addiction

To better understand the nature of habitual substance use, various models of addiction have been developed. Currently, the most popular model for understanding substance use disorders is to view them as diseases. Although this model has done much to lessen the stigma suffered by substance abusers and addicts and has resulted in more and improved treatment services, it is inadequate. It fails to address the importance of psychosocial and cognitive learning variables. A more useful means for understanding addiction is the motivated behavior model, as outlined in *The Perspectives of Psychiatry* by McHugh and Slavney.[1] This model properly takes into account the individual's free will, biological drive, and conditioned learning, all of which come together to produce addictive behavior.

Conditioned Learning

At the turn of the last century, several ideas explaining human behavior were prominent. Experimental behaviorists captured the imagination of much of the psychology field with their theory of learning. Pavlov showed that experiences linked to a particular stimulus, such as the ringing of a bell during a dog's feeding time, could cause the subject to behave a certain way in response to the stimulus, which in this case was the dog salivating at the sound of the bell.

Skinner elaborated on this on this work by developing the operant conditioning paradigm. Behaviors could be increased if they were followed immediately by rewards and decreased if followed immediately by punishment. In simple experiments, a monkey was conditioned to pull a lever to gain a food reward or to escape an electric shock. The more experience the animal has, the more frequently and readily it will pull the lever. This can be diagramed as in Fig. 5.1 and was called the *law of effect* by Thorndyke in 1913. He said essentially that the probability of a behavior can be increased or decreased, depending on its immediate consequence.

Skinner used this paradigm to investigate various factors that affect rates of behavior, which he termed *reinforcers*. Investigators in the 1970s and 1980s found that the liability to substance abuse and patterns of substance abuse can be modeled in this way. Addictive drugs not only will be self-administered, that is, animals will actively take the drugs if given an opportunity to do so, but also will reinforce self-administration; that is, animals will work (e.g., pull a lever, push a bar, peck a key) to gain access to the drugs.

This type of apparatus is illustrated in Fig. 5.2. In this apparatus, the animal sees a light go on. While it is illuminated, if the animal pulls the lever, food will be dispensed or drugs delivered. A baboon will pull the lever about 50–100 times to get banana-flavored pellets if he is hungry, about 500 times to get heroin if he is addicted, and about 5,000 times to get cocaine. In this experiment, we would say that cocaine is the most powerful reinforcer of lever-pulling behavior. A correlation exists between how many times an animal will pull the lever and the street

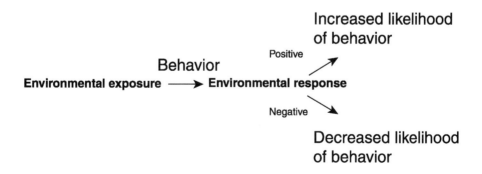

Fig. 5.1. Behavioral conditioning (behavioral learning)

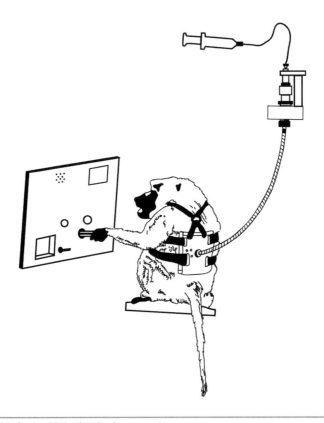

Fig. 5.2. Model of animal-behavior-shaping apparatus

value of a drug. Experiments of this type have led to a greater understanding of how the rewarding or reinforcing properties of drugs can shape behaviors.

A tight correlation exists between the reinforcing properties of drugs and their liability to addiction. One can measure the reinforcing properties of drugs by measuring how much work an animal will do to get the drug, how much discomfort the animal will tolerate to get the drug, and what the animal will give up to get the drug. As an example, one can teach animals that a particular lever will prevent an electric shock or provide access to food. One finds that animals will trade food and comfort for drugs, just as human addicts do routinely. In human drug addiction studies, we speak of the use-to-abuse ratio for drugs, which compares the number of people who use the drug with the number who become disordered by it. One in 20 is the commonly quoted figure for alcohol, while 1 in 3 is usually quoted for cocaine. The more reinforcing a drug is, the greater the likelihood of addiction.

Two other factors have been shown to influence drug use and abuse. The first is physical dependence, in which a drug administered over time will produce a state of physical withdrawal when it is stopped. The second is tolerance, in which a person will need increasing doses of the drug to produce the same effects as previously experienced at lower doses. Early models of addiction focused on tolerance and physical dependence as the most important factors in addiction. This led some researchers to the conviction that cocaine and amphetamines were not addictive, and later to the idea that addiction to them was a result of psychological dependence. It has become increasingly clear that reinforcement plays a critical role in driving behavior and addiction. Certain drugs cause addictions that do not produce physical dependence, but no addictive drug exists that does not reinforce behavior.

Conditioned learning shapes behavior by way of psychological and environmental responses to behavior. Society plays a role in shaping the choices involved in addiction, and alcoholism, for example, is far more prevalent than heroin dependence, in part because alcohol is legally available and drinking in moderation is culturally sanctioned. During Prohibition, the rates of alcoholism and alcohol-related morbidity sharply dropped. Learning is also shaped by both positive and negative reinforcement. In the early stages of addiction, the high or euphoria provided by the drug serves as the positive reinforcer. In the later stages, the addict develops physical dependence on the drug—he or she uses it to escape the withdrawal symptoms. When the reinforcer for the behavior is avoidance of a negative experience, the behavior paradigms call this *negative reinforcement*. (This differs from *punishment*, where a negative stimulus is applied after a behavior to decrease the frequency of the behavior.) Thus, long-term heroin addicts continue to use the drug not because it makes them high, but to avoid withdrawal sickness. As conditioned learning progresses, the behavior becomes more stereotypical and compulsive in nature.

The most important difference between most behaviors and the so-called motivated behaviors is the presence of an internal reward and drive. Many behaviors are conditioned by external factors such as the approval of parents and peers, status and material success, and, more directly, access to food, water, shelter, and other necessities. Certain activities, such as eating, sleeping, sexual activity, and drug use, are linked directly to the reward circuitry of brain. This causes people to develop appetites or drive states for these activities (we have heard patients describe their hunger for drugs). All these motivated behaviors are driven by visceral and neuroendocrine elements of reward and craving.

In the case of addiction, most substances of abuse have a strong effect on the mesolimbic dopaminergic system. This circuitry is located mainly in the midbrain, including the ventral tegmental area, the nucleus accumbens, and the medial forebrain bundle. The main neurotransmitter involved in this system is dopamine, but serotonin, norepinephrine, glutamate, and gamma-aminobutyric acid (GABA) are also important neurotransmitters. The mesolimbic structures are among the most primitive structures of the brain and affect behavior at its most fundamental level. For example, when animals are allowed to medicate themselves with substances of abuse, their behavior closely mimics those of humans. The driven, out-of-control feeling that addicts have about substances is in part mediated by the mesolimbic structures.

This is diagramed in Fig. 5.3. At the top of the figure is the external rein-forcement, but below we show the cycle of internal reinforcement associated with the positive feedback cycle of motivated behaviors. This cycle serves the purpose of amplifying behavior. Infants demonstrate this principle with the motivated behavior of eating. As they eat and receive an internal sense of reward, they gradually develop an increasing interest in eating. Although this behavior can become out of control, it is tightly regulated as an evolutionary safeguard, and one's appetite is shut off when he or she has had enough. The salience of behavior changes as well. Before eating, reading the menu is inter-esting, and one might even read about food that one would never really want, such as unusual dishes or things not to your own taste, but after dinner the menu has no salience, and reading it might even be faintly sickening. The turn-off or

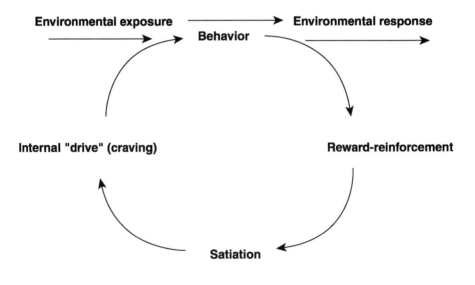

Fig. 5.3. The cycle of motivated behavior

inhibition of the feeding drive is activated after eating. When the turn-off is faulty, eating behavior can get out of control.

Positive feedback loops are inherently dangerous in biology. An important teleological question is why a positive feedback cycle that has the liability to get so out of control should be present. Its function is to amplify behaviors associated with survival. The internal rewards described previously are present only in important survival behaviors. Aversive experiences such as food poisoning will condition people not to eat anything even remotely like the food that made them sick, and this can result in a lifetime dislike of a particular food. Most people say immediately after getting food poisoning that they will never eat again. After a day or two, they will eat a little dry toast, and they get a sense of internal reward. The toast tastes good and provokes a strong, good feeling. This drives the desire to eat more foods and a gradual return to normal feeding. Feeding is necessary for survival, and the amplification cycle ensures that people will eventually eat again and that behaviors needed for survival will continue to occur. The power of this loop to condition behavior so that it will overcome even intensely aversive experiences is amply demonstrated by the resilience of behaviors such as eating, sleeping, drinking, and sexual activity.

The central issue for drug users is that, unlike feeding, sleeping, and sexual behaviors, addictive compounds were not present during the millions of years that this cycle took to evolve, and therefore the intrinsic turn-off mechanisms that are part of survival behaviors are not present for drug use. This makes the liability to substance use disorders higher and more dependent on exposure to positively reinforcing drugs than disorders of other motivated behaviors.

Given this description, why doesn't everyone become addicted? First of all, the cycle is inhibited and shaped by many factors. Protection against addiction can be shown to include close family and social structures, connections to others in the form of marital and social relationships, commitments to career and occupational life, and internalized structures such as religion and moral stances. All of these have been shown to protect individuals from addiction, and all inhibit the cycle shown earlier. They interfere with it taking control of life and to an extent immunize people against drug use disorders.

In fact, those that become dependent on substances and develop disorders associated with substance use are often in transitions during which the usual structure of life breaks down. The loss of a job and the breakup of a relationship are common concomitants of alcohol or drug use getting out of control. The patient may have always used a little too much alcohol, but now that he has lost his job he therefore does not need to get up in the morning. Also, a student leaving home for college may have no early classes and dramatically less supervision. A young person with a service job at McDonald's loses little if he is fired because he can be hired at another fast food restaurant. However, a person with a difficult-to-obtain position loses more if he is fired and therefore is relatively more protected from addiction, as his value of the job will impose limits on his behavior.

Other psychiatric and psychological factors also render persons more vulnerable, some of which are the central comorbidities of substance use disorders. The personality factors that make people more prone to taking risks also make them more likely to experiment with behaviors and, more sensitive to rewards. Extraverts are more sensitive to the reinforcing properties of drugs and less sensitive to the consequences of drug use; thus, they are at higher risk for addiction. Introverts are consequence and risk avoidant and are relatively protected from addiction. Depression makes the ordinary rewards of life less rewarding and increases people's sensitivity to the rewarding effects of drugs. Also, experiences that expose people to drugs and the social acceptance of drug use increase the risk of addiction.

Further, biology is involved in several ways. In the case of alcohol, genetic makeup affects the degree to which alcohol is rewarding. Some patients tell you that their first drink was so rewarding they began a lifetime of heavy drinking immediately. Others will say they never really liked drinking all that much and therefore were surprised that they became more and more dependent on alcohol to control the emotional discomforts of their lives. Cocaine is less affected by genetics, and patients with exposure to cocaine find it extremely rewarding, such that the use-to-abuse ratio is quite high. Other medical conditions such as chronic pain, a variety of disease states, and surgical procedures may result in exposure to addictive drugs. Such patients may develop iatrogenic addiction and then persistent drug use disorders. All these factors enhance or diminish the risk of the cycle getting out of control.

Finally, choice involves the free will of the individual to initiate and continue using the drug. Granted, one's choices become narrower as addiction progresses by way of stronger drives and conditioned learning, but only through an individual's choice can he or she enter treatment and change his or her lifestyle.

Categories of Substance Use Disorders

Substance use disorders span the spectrum of increasing use, dependence, and increasingly disordered functions. These stages often seem to blur together. It is often difficult to define precisely when the transition from heavy drinker to alcoholic occurs. Some persons use heavily but never actually become disordered by their use. Others are disordered by surprisingly modest use of a substance. The *Diagnostic and Statistical Manual of Mental Disorders* (DSM-IV)[2] divides disorders related to the use of psychoactive substances into two main categories: primary disorders of substance use and secondary substance-induced disorders. Substance use disorders include substance abuse and substance dependence.

Substance-induced disorders include substance intoxication, substance withdrawal, substance-induced psychotic disorders, substance-induced mood disorders, substance-induced anxiety disorders, substance-induced sleep disorders, substance-induced persisting dementia disorders, substance-induced amnestic disorders, and substance-induced sexual dysfunctions.

The criteria for substance dependence include tolerance or dependence. As stated earlier, tolerance refers to the need to use increasing amounts of the substance to achieve the same effect. Dependence is usually divided into two components: physiological and psychological. Physiological dependence occurs when the individual has physically adapted to the substance to the point that he or she must continue to use the substance to feel normal. If the individual stops using the substance abruptly, he or she experiences uncomfortable physical withdrawal symptoms, and the substance itself is used to prevent the individual from going into withdrawal. Psychological dependence occurs when the individual believes that he or she needs to continue using the substance to feel emotionally stable.

Substance abuse, on the other hand, is defined as a maladaptive pattern of using the substance that becomes socially, legally, or occupationally problematic for the individual. For example, a college student who becomes intoxicated at a fraternity party and misses a test the next day because he is sleeping off the effects of alcohol would demonstrate alcohol abuse, whereas the retired business executive who drinks martinis on a daily basis and suffers tremors and anxiety when he stops drinking would demonstrate alcohol dependence.

Substance Use Disorders and HIV Treatment

Ongoing substance use disorders have grave medical implications for HIV-infected individuals. Many physical symptoms of HIV infection overlap with those of substance abuse and dependence, including malaise, fatigue, weight loss, fevers, and night sweats. The accumulation of medical sequelae from chronic substance abuse accelerates the process of immunocompromise and amplifies the progressive burden of the HIV infection itself. IDUs, for example, are at higher risk for developing bacterial infections such as pneumonia, sepsis, soft tissue infections, and endocarditis. Tuberculosis, sexually transmitted diseases, hepatitis B and C, and coinfection with human T-cell lymphotrophic virus also occur more commonly in IDUs who are infected with HIV. Certain malignancies, lymphomas in particular, occur more frequently in HIV-infected drug users.

Neurologic symptoms can overlap between an HIV infection and substances of abuse. For instance, both AIDS dementia and drug intoxication can present with apathy, disorientation, aggression, and an altered level of consciousness. Withdrawal from alcohol and certain drugs can present with seizures and neurovegetative symptoms, as can opportunistic infections of the central nervous system (CNS). In addition, HIV-infected IDUs tend to be more at risk for developing fungal or bacterial infections of the brain and spinal cord.

Because the HIV-infected patient is likely to be on a variety of antiretroviral agents and prophylactic agents for opportunistic infections, the clinician must consider the interactions among these medications and the abused substances. Opioid users are at particular risk for medication interactions, such as the interaction between rifampin and methadone. Rifampin increases the elimination of methadone from the body and may result in the rapid onset of withdrawal symptoms in opiate addicts on maintenance therapy. This has important implications for treatment compliance in that the patient in a methadone program will be less likely to take his rifampin for fear of withdrawal. The antiviral medications can also have important interactions with opiates. Ritonavir, for example, increases the serum levels of opiates in the body. HIV medications such as didanosine (ddI, Videx, Videx EC) may also cause peripheral neuropathies, which may be worsened by the neurotoxic effects of alcohol, vitamin deficiency, and malnutrition related to chronic substance abuse.

Assessment and Evaluation

Patient History

Because of the societal stigma attached to both substance abuse and HIV, the patient may be reluctant to disclose information. Forming a close therapeutic alliance is the first step in effective assessment and treatment. The clinician should take a nonjudgmental and empathetic approach to interviewing the patient. Confidentiality should be assured as in other types of medical settings. In many cases, collateral sources of information can be helpful in eliciting accurate histories. These may include old medical records, family members, friends, and health care providers.

A substance use history should contain specific information about not only the substances used but also the methods of administration, duration, frequency of use, most recent use, and amount used of each drug. The patient should also be asked about periods of abstinence, relapse, and the respective conditions favoring each one.

A drug treatment history should also be obtained, including the types and period of detoxification, outpatient drug treatment, and residential drug treatment. This information is helpful in ascertaining which methods of treatment may have been helpful in the past and which treatment modalities have failed.

To assess for drug dependency, questions related to drug craving, the triggers for drug usage, withdrawal symptoms, medical complications, and impaired psychosocial functioning should be discussed. Particular psychosocial problems related to drug use include marital and family problems, lack of employment, homelessness, and legal difficulties. A variety of clinician-based methods to screen for substance abuse have been developed, the most commonly cited is the CAGE questionnaire. This consists of the following four questions:

- Have you ever tried to _cut_ down?
- Have you become _annoyed_ when others talk about your drinking?
- Have you ever had _guilt_ over your substance use?
- Have you ever had an _eye opener_?

A "yes" answer to two of these questions indicates problem use, but we recommend using these questions as a starting point for a more in-depth conversation, rather than as a comprehensive screening tool in themselves.

Physical Examination

A complete physical examination should include a careful search for physical evidence of drug use, including injection marks, scars, burns, nasal septum erosion or perforation, skin abscesses, cellulitis, and soft-tissue infection. Signs of chronic alcohol abuse include spider angiomata on the chest and abdomen, reddened palms, testicular atrophy, ascites, hepatosplenomegaly, and physical trauma. A careful neurologic assessment, including a complete mental status examination, is essential to assess for the presence of both substance intoxication and the neuropsychiatric manifestations of AIDS.

Laboratory Studies

In addition to HIV antibody testing, patients should have a complete blood count, chemistry profile, liver profile, hepatitis B and C serology, and rapid plasma reagin to test for syphilis. CD4 counts and viral loads should be checked on a regular basis to monitor the progression of HIV infection. Serum and urine toxicology screens can be useful in ascertaining recent drug use, as well as evaluating patients who display any acute change in mental status.

Co-occurring Psychiatric Disorders

The term _dual diagnosis_ refers to a patient who has both a substance use disorder and another psychiatric malady. A _triple diagnosis_ usually refers to a dual-diagnosis patient who also has HIV. Such patients are overrepresented in treatment settings because of their symptom severity and chronicity. For instance, in inner-city Baltimore, as many as 44 percent of new entrants to the

HIV medical clinic at Johns Hopkins Hospital have an active substance use disorder. Twenty-four percent of these patients have both a current substance abuse disorder and another non-substance-related Axis I diagnosis.

Difficulties in the realm of personality are among the most common psychiatric problems seen in this population. Although personality disorder diagnoses are currently described in a categorical fashion in the DSM-IV, it is probably more useful to view personality as dimensional in nature. Using this model, personality traits exist along a continuum that predicts habitual maladaptive approaches to life's difficulties.

In Chapter 4, we described a dimensional model of temperament, one of the major components of personality. This model depicts temperament as existing around the axes of stability/instability and introversion/extraversion. The combination of instability and extraversion is often seen in patients being treated in the HIV clinic. Persons with extreme traits of instability have very strong and reactive emotional responses that tend to be overpowering, easily taking over the persons' judgment and behavior. Additionally, persons who are extreme extraverts have emotional responses that are very quick and changeable, as they are focused in the present (rather than the past or future). These persons tend to seek rewards rather than avoid harm.

Unstable extraversion has important implications for the HIV-positive addict. These traits not only result in a vulnerability to addiction and other risky behaviors that predispose one to become infected with HIV, but they also pose significant barriers to treatment. These patients tend to act on strong, impulsive feelings rather than on carefully considered treatment instructions. Their behavior will often be driven by the transient, immediate rewards of drugs rather than by their lasting future consequences. Such patients tend to become bored easily and treatment is often unexciting. They "want what they want when they want it," rather than when it may be good for them. It is critical to identify these personality vulnerabilities in this patient population because they can have a profound effect on treatment engagement and prognosis.

Affective (mood) disorders are also commonly found in these patients. Diagnosing such disorders (and other psychiatric disorders) in drug users can be difficult and even controversial. The controversy stems from the problem in determining the causal, or even chronological, relationship between drug disorders and affective disorders. Although some theorists have wanted to emphasize the primacy of one or the other in guiding treatment, this "chicken or egg" approach is not especially productive. Given the high prevalence of overlapping addictive and affective disorders in clinical settings, as well as the very poor prognosis associated with untreated affective disorders, a treatment approach should emphasize simultaneous and equal treatment of both entities. This is not to suggest that it is easy to distinguish transient depressive symptoms caused by drug withdrawal from symptoms caused by demoralization or from persistent depressive symptoms that indicate a major affective disorder. It often becomes necessary to observe the patient over a period of abstinence in a confined treatment setting before this can be elucidated. Facts from the patient's clinical history may also be supportive of an affective disorder diagnosis.

It is important to identify affective disorders not only to avoid their well-known sequelae, including suicide, but also because of their complex interactions with addiction. Depression is associated with the worsening of addiction and a resistance to treatment. The anhedonia of depression makes it difficult for addicts to respond to and enjoy life's other rewards. Depressed patients also find it more difficult to engage, invest in, and sustain treatment given their apathy and negativism. It is essential, therefore, for the clinician to recognize and treat depression early to maximize a successful treatment outcome.

Treatment

Although oversimplified, the steps for the treatment of substance use disorders can be outlined in the following way. Several of these steps may occur simultaneously as treatment begins, and some may be repeated or ongoing while working on others, but here we will describe them as a sequence. Essential issues in the treatment of substance use disorders can be summarized as follows:

- Induction of patient role
- Detoxification
- Treatment of comorbid conditions
- Rehabilitation
- Prevention of relapse

Role Induction and Motivation to Change

The initial and often most daunting task of treating an addict is engagement and induction of the patient role. The general rule is that addicts and treatment providers begin with differing agendas. Addicts tend to come to the treatment setting seeking comfort and crisis relief, whereas physicians and other health care providers look at the long-term goal of improving the patient's health and function. One of the critical initial tasks the health provider faces is that of persuasion. The addict must come to the realization that his or her agenda is actually the same as that of the treatment team.

Many authors, most notably Prochaska and DiClemente,[3] have described a "transtheoretical stages of change" model to elucidate the addiction and recovery process. The patient is viewed as progressing through several different stages of change in the recovery process:

1. Precontemplation: The patient has no intention to change his or her addictive behavior.
2. Contemplation: The patient considers change because of the negative consequences of his or her drug use but is ambivalent about it.
3. Preparation: The patient shows an intent to change and takes the initial steps to seek treatment.
4. Action: The patient decides to modify his or her behavior, environment, and circumstances in order to relinquish the addictive lifestyle.
5. Maintenance: The patient works to prevent a relapse and consolidate his or her changed behavior and lifestyle.

The most difficult task faced by clinicians is preparing and moving the patient from a contemplative stage to an action stage. A technique known as *motivational interviewing* described by Miller and Rollnick[4] facilitates the patient's readiness to change. It uses empathy and gentle confrontation to amplify the discrepancy between the substance abuser's current lifestyle and his or her long-term, life-enhancing goals.

Detoxification

For intoxicated patients to understand and process the cognitive steps needed for recovery, detoxification is the first step. Many HIV-positive substance abusers benefit from a brief hospital stay to stabilize their psychiatric and medical comorbidities. Slowly tapering either the drug of dependence or using a cross-dependent drug that has a similar pharmacologic mechanism of action best accomplishes detoxification.

Detoxification is often unpleasant, and no evidence supports the idea that noxious withdrawal during detoxification improves one's outcome. In fact, some behavioral studies suggest that patients suffering through severe withdrawal may actually develop conditioned withdrawal such that exposure to environments similar to the one experienced during "cold turkey withdrawal" can bring withdrawal symptoms back months later.

Benzodiazepine, barbiturate, and alcohol withdrawal can be life threatening. Active tapers, which use a slowly decreased dose of drug from the class to which the patient is addicted, may be used for opiates and sedative-hypnotics. Drugs such as dicyclomine (Bentyl), prochlorperazine (Compazine), promethazine (Phenergan), methocarbamol (Robaxin), and clonidine (Catapres) can ameliorate the unpleasant symptoms of withdrawal. We use these liberally during tapers of opiate- and sedative-hypnotic-addicted patients. A debate surrounds whether to use active tapers when it is not necessary and whether to taper slowly or rapidly. Additionally, an active debate is taking place about how long to leave patients on drugs that are useful for tapering off addictive compounds. We have used clonidine for years for some of our patients. Although clonidine is not particularly reinforcing for patients who have not taken opiates, it is somewhat reinforcing for opiate-experienced patients, has some street value to opiate addicts, and is sold illicitly by some patients.

Some authors have used antidepressants to help patients taper from psychomotor stimulant classes of drugs (amphetamines and cocaine), but data to support such practices are controversial. We tend to reserve this for patients whose symptoms of major depression are clearly present.

Alcohol and other sedative-hypnotic agents should be detoxified through the use of an active taper, as they can produce a life-threatening withdrawal syndrome. Most can be tapered with a substituted agent from this class. The most common tapers use a benzodiazepine such as diazepam (Valium), chlordiazepoxide (Librium), lorazepam (Ativan), or oxazepam (Serax). We favor the use of long half-life drugs such as diazepam. Some authors recommend the use of drugs that are minimally metabolized by the liver such as oxazepam and lorazepam, particularly in advanced alcohol abuse, as these patients may have compromised liver functions. Some drugs are particularly difficult to taper. The drugs alprazolam (Xanax), triazolam (Halcion), and clonazepam (Klonopin) may be particularly difficult to taper and seem to substitute for each other better than other sedative-hypnotic agents, and we have found that clonazepam may be the best long-acting drug to use for these tapers. Some patients actually require the drug they were using for the most rapid and least uncomfortable taper. The drug clorazepate (Tranxene) may also be particularly difficult to detoxify in some patients and may be better tapered without substitution.

The detoxification of opiates is accomplished through a substituted taper of long-acting opioid agonists such as methadone. Alternative agents that can be used include buprenorphine, a mixed opioid agonist-antagonist and clonidine, an alpha-2 agonist, which can bring symptomatic relief of heroin withdrawal. A good deal of debate exists over how gently to taper these drugs, whether they need to be used only on an inpatient basis, how much clonidine to use, and whether or not opiate addicts all need methadone maintenance (see the following section) or if some can be drug-free after a taper.

Treatment of Comorbid Psychiatric Conditions

As stated earlier, many patients with HIV and addictions often have comorbid psychiatric conditions that need to be treated in order to maximize compliance and abstinence. Conditions such as major depression, bipolar disorder, and schizophrenia are best managed with pharmacologic treatments. Because these patients tend to have multiple medical complications, it is important to remember to start medications at low dosages and to titrate slowly in order to minimize the risk of developing adverse side effects and delirium.

Disorders of personality, in particular unstable extroversion, are managed with psychotherapy. The ways that unstable extroverts may sabotage treatment include staff splitting (pitting staff members against each other by manipulation), doctor shopping, general noncompliance, and manipulative behavior. Therapy addressing these personality issues should include firm limit-setting and a devotion to consistency on the part of all the health care providers involved. To this end, it is essential to have a documented treatment plan that clearly states the goals agreed on by all the staff. The treatment plan should be reviewed with the patients at the initiation of treatment so that they understand clearly what is expected of them and what they can expect from the treatment providers if they adhere to the goals.

Maintenance Treatment and Relapse Prevention

After detoxification, the treatment of comorbid conditions, and role induction are accomplished, long-term treatment is necessary for patients to begin the process of lifestyle change and recovery. Because this patient population is complicated and especially vulnerable to recidivism, one must take an integrated approach to treatment. To this end, a one-stop shopping model is especially useful for maintaining treatment progress. Thus, a treatment center catering to HIV-positive addicts should ideally include medical providers, psychiatrists, social workers, housing counselors, and day care workers in addition to substance abuse counselors. This integrated approach will help to bring order out of these patients' chaotic lifestyles.

It is important to remember that addiction treatment is active rather than passive and entails transforming previously held beliefs, attitudes, and personal identity into a new way of life. To this end, group therapy is a necessary part of all substance use disorder treatment, whether it be one of the 12-step models, network therapy, rational recovery, therapeutic community, or the many other models of recovery currently practiced. In group therapy, the most experienced members of the group provide both confrontation and support for the newly initiated member. Group support also provides the newly recovering addict with a hopeful view of the benefits to be achieved with recovery. A commitment to a recovery group protects the patient from the influences of the drug community and provides the patient with new bonds that help maintain a sense of purpose and hope.

Therapy should include a focus on identifying triggers to substance use, minimizing or decreasing exposure to substances, and defining a clear plan for relapse prevention. It is important to realize that relapse is often the rule and not the exception, and plans should be in place for early intervention in case of relapse. Monitoring measures such as urine checks, serum toxicologies, and Breathalyzer tests can help monitor success. Contingency management, using a variety of positive and negative reinforcers tied to urine toxicology results, has also been shown to be highly effective in maintaining sobriety.

Individual and family therapies can enhance the effectiveness of treatment but should not take the place of group therapy. In individual treatment, it is important that the treatment provider remain flexible in his or her treatment approach. Thus, a cognitive-behavioral approach may work for some patients, whereas others may do better with a modified psychodynamic approach.

Pharmacologic treatments should be seen as enhancements to the overall treatment plan and not as a sole therapy. In a sense, it is an adjunctive treatment. Certain people are advocates for the idea that if patients are engaged in adequate pharmacologic therapy, they will rehabilitate themselves, and this remains a subject of research and debate. We contend that, given a choice between more treatment or less, we tend to choose more. Pharmacologic treatment can be divided into the categories shown in Table 5.1.

All the interventions described have been supported by some studies. A relapse can occur impulsively, and some patients are eager for a type of insur-

Table 5.1. Pharmacologic adjuncts for the treatment of addiction

- Aversive conditioning
  - Disulfiram (alcohol)
- Blockade of reinforcement
  - Naltrexone (opioids)
- Drive suppression
  - Bupropion (tobacco)
  - Buprenorphine (cocaine)
  - Naltrexone (alcohol, tobacco?)
- Substituted addiction
  - Methadone, LAAM, Buprenorphine (opioids)

ance so that they will not blow it in a single weak moment. They have often had experience with this in the past and know their weak moments. Drugs like disulfiram (an inhibitor of acetaldehyde dehydrogenase) can be very effective. The alcohol contained in alcoholic beverages is ethanol, which is metabolized in two steps. In the first step, the ethanol is catalyzed by the enzyme alcohol dehydrogenase, which makes acetaldehyde, a highly toxic substance responsible for many of the unpleasant effects of intoxication. This is then broken down to acetic acid (vinegar) by a second enzyme, aldehyde dehydrogenase. Disulfiram (Antabuse) inhibits this enzyme and makes people ill by causing high levels of acetaldehyde. It is taken once daily at dosages from 250 mg to 500 mg and causes an unpleasant reaction when alcohol is ingested because of the buildup of acetaldehyde in the body. Symptoms include nausea, facial flushing, headaches, and hypotension. Liver enzymes should be monitored because of the risk of hepatatoxicity. Importantly, several commonly used medicines cause disulfiram-like reactions because they inhibit acetaldehyde dehydorgenase. Patients who are prescribed such medicines, like metronidazole (Flagyl, an antibiotic), should be warned of this reaction so as not to have unpleasant effects. We have also known doctors who have prescribed metronidazole to patients with alcohol problems for its disulfiram-like effects. We do not encourage this practice, as chronic metronidazole use may be complicated by the development of resistant bacterial strains colonizing the patient. The practice also conveys something telling about the practitioner's reluctance to discuss disulfiram prescription directly, which may be a significant barrier to the patient's recovery.

Naltrexone is an opioid antagonist that has a high affinity for blocking opiate receptors, making it difficult to impossible to experience opiate reinforcement. The discovery of opiate receptors and opiate blockers has given great hope that these compounds can help in preventing heroin and morphine abuse. Naloxone is effective only in a injected form, but naltrexone is effective orally. Taking naltrexone effectively blocks all the receptors for opiates. It is surprising how few effects opiate antagonists cause in opiate-naive subjects. This is in stark contrast to the overwhelming withdrawal caused by the administration of these agents to physically dependent subjects, who have an acute onset of catastrophic withdrawal.

After effective detoxification, patients can take naltrexone, and while it is present, they cannot experience an opiate high at even substantial doses of narcotics. This means that daily usage of naltrexone can effectively prevent a patient from returning to opiate use. The problem is that in clinical practice few patients will take it regularly enough for it to be effective. We are awaiting a naltrexone formula that can be given as a sustained release medication that is effective over time. Naltrexone can be taken orally once daily at dosages ranging from 50 to

100 mg. As with disulfiram, liver function tests are monitored in patients on naltrexone because of the risk of hepatotoxicity.

Several drugs have been shown to reduce the drive or craving for other seemingly unrelated compounds. The antidepressant bupropion (Wellbutrin)
decreases cravings for nicotine and appears to be much less toxic. At 300 mg
each day, it improves the outcome of smoking cessation programs. Naltrexone
has been shown to reduce alcohol cravings across a number of studies.
Buprenorphine and some antidepressants may reduce the cravings for cocaine.

The most controversial and well studied treatment option is called agonist
substitution (methadone maintenance is an example). In this approach, the reinforcing properties of a class of drugs are used to positively condition patients
toward rehabilitation, behavioral control, and abstinence from the use of illicit
drugs. The biggest controversy involves the fact that although these patients are
demonstrably more functional, they remain addicted to the drugs used for maintenance. The approach involves the daily administration of long-acting, high
doses of an agonist from the class of drugs to which the patient is addicted. The
success of the approach is dependent on the ability to develop a tolerance to the
effects of the drugs and therefore to become increasingly functional despite high
doses of medication.

The most common form of agonist substitution is methadone maintenance
for heroin addiction. Methadone is given at high doses, and over time patients
become tolerant to its effects. Because the methadone is given at 3–10 times the
amount of opiate that most heroin addicts use, patients are unaffected by street
doses of heroin and therefore have little motivation to use it. In addition to
meeting behavior goals, patients come for daily treatment, which includes gradually increasing doses of methadone that range from 40 to 200 mg each day. The
medication is administered under supervision until the patient has established a
pattern of abstinence. At this point, take-home dosages are often allowed. The
best programs combine occupational, vocational, and social rehabilitation, as
well as a reintegration program to support and stabilize relapse prevention. A
good program would also screen for other drugs and treat patients for other
addictions. Some programs have integrated HIV care with methadone main-
tainance with striking success in terms of adherence and treatment outcome.

A newer partial agonist, buprenorphine, has been approved for oral administration and may be a useful alternative to methadone. The latest initiative for
treating opiate addiction is the use of outpatient buprenorphine for opiate agonist maintenance. The drug occupies the opiate receptors but causes less intoxication than heroin or methadone. If the patient uses heroin while on
buprenorphine, he or she does not experience any intoxication because of the
tightness of buprenorphine binding to the receptors. Additionally, although

buprenorphine tablets can be ground up and injected, a new formulation of buprenorphine combined with naloxone is now being made available. If taken orally, the naloxone is inactive, but if injected it blocks opiate receptors and causes withdrawal. In the studies so far, this prevents injection abuse of the drug and allows for better oral maintenance.

It is clear that methadone maintenance decreases illicit drug use, crime, and drug-related morbidity and mortality, as well as improves the functioning of patients. It can be argued, however, that patients on methadone are still less functional than those who are medication free. It can also be argued that such people are still addicted and therefore not truly "free" in a metaphysical sense. Methadone maintenance is also much less expensive than addiction, but more expensive than other treatment options.

In what we consider to be an unfortunate choice of terminology, methadone maintenance is often included in a group of treatments called "harm-reduction" treatments. The idea behind these treatments is that the patient is harmed less by the treatment than by the original behavior. Although this is true, it is also true that methadone maintenance can improve functioning, quality of life, and longevity—goals for treatment we have found worth making explicit to patients. The use of substituted benzodiazepine maintenance for alcoholics has been less popular as it is hard to demonstrate that these patients are more functional than alcoholics.

This methadone debate is part of a larger argument about the issues of treatment as opposed to criminal punishment and about the legalization of illicit drugs. Many people describe drug use as a choice, as if it were a free choice. Although it is true that many patients stop using drugs despite the biological nature of addiction, we have yet to encounter a patient who chooses to be an addict. People choose to use drugs, always believing they can quit using if they wish to, because they have never encountered anything as sneaky and foul as addiction. Each turn of the behavioral cycle makes it more difficult to resist using drugs, but not impossible. Then the person discovers the craving, gnawing need, the sense of "can't" that addicts have. Good clinicians help them to see the difference between "can't" and "won't" and free them from the prison of their feelings. Although every study shows that treatment saves money, it is not the fundamental reason to treat addictions. It is because treatment is the right thing to do. Drug addiction brings misery and suffering to everyone it touches.

As for legalization, it depends on the ratio of good to harm for a particular drug. Most arguments about the legalization of drugs focus on illegal drugs without discrimination among them. These discussions include drugs like marijuana in the same category as drugs like amphetamine. Legalizing a drug like marijuana, where the use-to-abuse ratio is probably less than for alcohol, is a different matter than legalizing cocaine, which has a use-to-abuse ratio of about one in three. Making alcohol illegal in the early 1900s led to organized crime, a wholesale disregard for the law, and the virtual disappearance of alcoholic liver disease. One must trade benefits and risks in the decision to legalize a pharmacologic agent, but one must distinguish between different drugs. Cocaine has a use-to-abuse ratio such that one out of three users will develop serious difficulties related to usage, the highest use-to-abuse ratio of any drug investigated. The ratios for amphetamines and other psychomotor stimulants range close to cocaine, opiates slightly less at one 1 of 9, and alcohol least at 1 out of 20. Data for marijuana and other compounds without a demonstrable physical dependence syndrome are less clear, but they may approximate alcohol or be even lower. Vulnerable people, adolescents, people with depression, and some people with genetic loading for addiction are at increased risk. A plan to legalize drugs needs to address these issues and decide which drugs should be legalized.

As health care providers, we like to point out that we advocate for health, and the risk of addictive drug use is often much higher than the demonstrable health care benefit. We quote the wisdom of Paul McHugh, who said of substance use and addiction, "I'll take less." We could do with less addiction and drug use, less alcoholism, and less tobacco use. On the other hand, if we wish to allow people to use these substances legally, we must provide adequate treatment for those vulnerable people who become trapped in addictions, or we have done more harm than good.

Case: Substance Abuse and Depression

E is a 47-year-old white man who was originally seen with his wife for couples therapy, depression, and addiction. During his initial interview, he complained that his wife was supporting her addiction by working as a prostitute and that he "couldn't take it any more."

E's family history includes depression and alcoholism in several relatives, including his mother. He had no delays in early development but was diagnosed with severe dyslexia in the fourth grade. He graduated from high school and had some college education. Although E was quite intelligent, his academic performance was uneven because of his dyslexia. He has been married three times and has six children, all of whom were in foster care. At the time of his initial evaluation, he was desperately trying to keep the children he had with his third wife, and this was a large part of his early motivation for treatment.

E's mother initially exposed him to alcohol when he was a child by giving it to him to help him sleep. He began to drink heavily in his early teens and would drink excessively in binges from that time on. At age 14, he began to use amphetamines and other stimulants, which became his drugs of choice for much of his life. He started using intravenous heroin in his twenties, although he denied he was addicted until his third marriage, when his heroin use with his wife came to occupy most of his time. He has used cocaine and other drugs, including using marijuana regularly.

E has received disability income for his dyslexia and bipolar illness intermittently throughout his life. He has worked at many different jobs, including work as a drug addiction counselor, a psychiatric nursing aide, and a security guard. He was involved in motorcycle clubs and a variety of illegal activities related to the clubs. His first clear symptoms of psychiatric illness began in his teens but received little attention until his treatment with us. He has a long history of HIV disease, hepatitis B and C, alcoholic liver disease, cervical spinal fractures related to a motor vehicle accident, hypertension, gonorrhea, syphilis, chlamydia, and other sexually transmitted diseases.

E presented complaining of sadness, intense irritability, and a wish that he could just die. His sleep and appetite were poor. He had a global loss of pleasure and reported he had not had fun in years. On several occasions he had tried to kill himself by deliberate heroin overdose in the throes of despair over his situation. The thing that bothered him most was that his wife occasionally brought customers into their house and used their bed to turn tricks. He stated that he needed to get straight to take care of his kids and that on several occasions he had stopped using heroin by barring his wife from their house while she was using. He reported that when he stopped drugs she would tell him about her sexual liaisons with other men to make him jealous, and he would feel compelled to let her come home, where she would seduce him with sex and drugs.

During their initial interview, E's wife agreed that this was indeed the pattern that had developed. She stated that he did an adequate job of caring for the children and that his disability check paid for part of their drug use, but that she needed either to work or to prostitute to gain enough money for drugs. She suggested that he could also sell drugs, but then he would not be home to care for the children. She thought that at times his temper made it dangerous for her to be around him, but she admitted that this was also part of the excitement of their life together. She mentioned that he had become violent with her when he was jealous and that the police had come to their home over domestic disputes.

E was quite aware of his addiction. He admitted that he had been addicted all his life to something, including drugs, alcohol, and destructive women. In the initial interview, he stated that he hated groups and would not go to group treatment. We told him that he was not required to *like* group therapy, but he was required simply to *attend*. We added that most treatment in medicine is unpleasant, but that his condition was similar to treatable cancer for which many patients undergo surgery, chemotherapy, and/or radiation. He did not attempt to argue that he was doing well without treatment. E was more willing to consider treatment than his wife, but both initially engaged in treatment with the HIV team. E was significantly sicker, with liver disease that limited his treatment options to some extent.

He attended group treatments, stopped drinking and using amphetamines, but he relapsed to heroin whenever his wife began to use again herself. She would relapse and resume working as a prostitute, causing E to relapse as well. This cycle occurred repeatedly over the next several years. They became seriously delinquent in rent payments and E owed a large amount of child support for his other children. Social services had become involved in an effort to protect their children and were visiting regularly, threatening to remove the children to foster care.

E had severe chronic back and neck pain as well as depression and was initially admitted to the inpatient service for detoxification and the initiation of antidepressant therapy. He began treatment with fluoxetine with very limited improvement in his mood. Several trials of other antidepressants failed to improve his depression. After his first discharge from the hospital, the cycles described earlier began. E did quite well on desipramine, which helped his depression, chronic pain, concentration, appetite, and sleep.

Unfortunately, E's wife continued to play a destructive role in his life. At one point, she was discharged from the inpatient service when she was caught exchanging sex for drugs with other patients. Later she was discharged from the HIV clinic for illegal activities on the premises. She was repeatedly arrested, and each time E would allow her back into the house with the same results. Finally, during one of E's inpatient stays, we discussed the fact that we could not watch him continue to self-destruct and that it was time to give up his destructive relationship with his wife. We pointed out that he might be playing a role in enabling his wife to use drugs because he was a source of money and a place to stay, and thus a way for her to avoid the consequences of her behavior. About this time, his children were removed from his home and placed in foster care. He agreed to separate from his wife when this happened, saying that he would kill himself unless he got his children back and that they were all he had to live for.

He returned two months later, having done quite well, and said that he was unable to give up his wife and asked for one more chance to work with us while trying to live with her. We reluctantly agreed but told E we thought there was no chance he could remain sober with her while she used heroin. He bet us that he would be able to do it this time, and he remained sober, attending groups and working hard at his sobriety. His wife continued to use heroin, but at this point it began to drive him away from her. He remained sober despite several episodes of depression and his difficult situation at home. His CD4 cell count fell to nearly 200 and he began HIV treatment with a highly active antiretroviral therapy (HAART) regimen. After two years of sobriety, he came to us and told us he was separating from his wife, saying "Even I can't take it anymore."

E continued in therapy, working on issues of his failed relationships, his patterns of addiction, and his craving to reunite with his wife. He began to develop several hobbies and become involved in AIDS activism. He did peer counseling with heterosexual patients who were struggling with AIDS, and he founded a successful program and a support network directed at heterosexual people with HIV. One of his hobbies has developed into a small, home-based specialty business that has been successful. He continues to be followed in our clinic, maintains a close relationship with his therapist, and continued to struggle with his estranged wife's efforts to draw him back into her life. As of this writing, however, his wife has died of a drug overdose. E has grieved for some months, but maintains sobriety and continues antidepressant medication and psychotherapy.

Discussion

This is a case of severe addiction in a person imbedded in an addictive life. E's addiction has created the circumstances he is in, including poverty, desperation, and a need to focus on just getting through each day. On the other hand, his life also contributed to his addiction by constantly thwarting efforts to change, leading him back to the same people and places, and creating insurmountable obstacles that demoralized him completely.

E is a good example of many issues. The recognition of "hitting rock bottom," as described in recovery circles, did not occur for E until he lost his children and saw his wife in their bed with a customer working as a prostitute. E resisted the recovery motto of changing "people, places, and things" until the evidence of the necessity to do so became completely clear to him. Help and guidance, particularly in the form of direction from his therapist, was very difficult for him to accept. Finally, commitment to group treatment, discovery of a spiritual power, and conversion to active relapse prevention were very difficult for him.

This case also illustrates the strength of the person who can survive addiction. Many people lack the necessary resilience to overcome their losses and restart their lives. E made a good addict because he is able to focus on one day at a time, and he engaged in recovery by using the same "one day at a time" approach (another catchphrase in the recovery world). He is charming, an endowment he used to manipulate others while he was addicted but that is also useful in keeping his health care providers from giving up despite seemingly endless failures. We liked him and wanted to save his life, even though we knew he had done some terrible things.

As we describe in Chapter 5, E needed all the elements of a well-thought-out drug addiction treatment plan to succeed: induction into the patient role, detoxification, the treatment of comorbid depression and personality vulnerabilities, rehabilitation, and the ongoing prevention of a relapse. His remarkable recovery belongs to him. The number of failures in the world of addiction treatment speaks to the fact that it is not the doctor, the program, or the medication that makes addiction treatment successful, but the patient's commitment to continue the treatment despite its difficulties.

Patient's Commentary

"To get to the beginning of my illness and my addiction (a.k.a. that big hairy monster that lived on my back), it started early in a Puerto Rican and Irish American who was different in the world of the late 1950s and '60s. I lived in two worlds, one a strong Hispanic one, and kept that as a secret. When I entered school, it was found that I had dyslexia though I had a high IQ. I can't read very well. This put me in the slow classes, where I was bored to death. Let's say I was mocked as soon as I opened my mouth. When Woodstock and the drug craze came in, it didn't take long for me to start. At that time there was a smorgasbord of drugs where I lived. Drugs made me popular, I thought. I could get girls, oh yes, my other addiction. I was a codependent. I felt that I needed a woman on my arm to fulfill my sense of self. My drug usage became a regular part of my day, but things increasingly got worse as the years wore on and as the decades passed.

"When I met my third wife, my two addictions crashed and I lost total control. She introduced me to IV heroin and cocaine, and the genie was out of the bottle. We were spending $200 and drinking a fifth of Jack Daniels a day. This took a lot of work to do. We worked all night and day stealing and hustling, we were always fighting about drugs, and we both were constantly getting locked up. We had four children and I tried to keep them going. I took care of them the best I could and took them to school and church, but drugs ruled the house. This love for my children was one of my catalysts for change.

"I found out that I was HIV positive and I became deeply depressed and increased the use of street drugs. I couldn't stop yet. It was truly amazing that I didn't drown there. I was isolated from my family and friends. My life was entwined in this sick, codependent marriage. Two addicts can't live normal lives. I would get drunk and then fighting was part of our script, often violent with all control lost. I kept getting locked up. My wife was a violent woman and was my downfall. I would get locked up for my impaired judgment. I would react poorly. I would not run but would fight or I would steal something or be in the wrong place at the wrong time.

"After one time in jail after I was placed in treatment, someone said, 'Have you had enough?' And this time I had. The strange thing is HIV changed me. I had the opportunity to enter regular treatment. I did not quit treatment this time, even though I still was using for part of this time. But the treatment team stayed there this time. Wow, I was surprised. I felt I had value. They listened. Most people had long ago stopped, including myself, but I wanted more now. Somehow I had a light to go on. I had started on psychiatric meds. I cleaned up some. I tried this to do it on my own for me, not court imposed. This time I was the catalyst of my own change. I stated that 'I quit' and I did.

"Well, it was not that easy. I was living in a basement with a house full of people getting high. I stayed downstairs and kicked, and it hurt like hell, but I stuck it out. I used clonidine and lived through the pain. The pain I felt gave me resolve to stay off the shit. I wish I could say all things became well, but life can't be that way. I needed to go into the hospital, so I put my kids in foster care and started a long period of hospitalization. I was deeply depressed. I missed, I missed. I had quit. I was growing and that was as painful to me as withdrawal. There was a long cycle of hospital treatment and day hospital treatment, and all the while I saw my therapy team and tried to keep in contact with my kids, but the state kept them. We were headed to court and were losing this battle. I won't dwell on this, but my heart was broken but I chose not to pick up. This was a real change, but I won't write any more on this.

"My marriage is another story. I was still codependent. I was growing, but my wife wasn't. She still wanted drugs, and this caused much fighting, but I was still trying to save her. That was my need. I was still addicted to her. I finally saw this and 4 1/2 years into my recovery I ended my marriage and had my wife removed from our house. For the first time in a decade, I was free of my monster. I learned that I was all right. I could let go of my resentments and my addictions.

"In looking at my life then and now, I can see several differences. The main one is that I don't feel a need to escape from myself. I have learned to turn away from those voices that caused me to be filled with self-doubt. I don't need the validation of others to make me feel good about myself.

"I have been a patient at Johns Hopkins since 1987. [My therapist] has been a blessing. I really respect her because she has gone beyond her duty in seeing that I get the best treatment I could get. I have manic depression. When I came to Johns Hopkins, I was very sick. My doctors saved my life, never giving up on me. They have really helped me with my sickness. They know how to prescribe my medications for me to get well. They are wonderful at what they do.

"I decided to put my past behind with the help of my doctors and move on to the future. I have worked on family issues, learning to let go of some of the pain I have lived with since I was a child. I had been under the care of [another doctor] and he changed my medicine, and I ended up on the psychiatric ward because I became psychotic. My father died in March of 1999 and my son died on January 18, 2000. I had a lot of therapy to help me deal with my losses. I got very depressed and was put in the hospital for treatment. When I got out of the hospital, I went back for psychotherapy. It was very scary when they changed my medicine and started all over again.

"Psychotherapy has really been a blessing for me. My therapist always knows when I am getting depressed and need to make a change with my medications or even be hospitalized. Sometimes it is very hard to be patient with the change in my medications. Sometimes I just get so psychotic it takes a while to get better. I have been very sick and confused in the past, and my psychotherapist works very hard to bring me back to a good state of mind. I trust in her. Psychotherapy was the beginning of my life, helping me heal from my past and deal with the present. I want to thank the psychiatric staff at Johns Hopkins for saving my life. They have never given up on me, nor will I ever give up on myself."

Chapter Six
Sexual Problems and HIV

The medical concepts regarding sexual disorders have undergone much criticism and rethinking over the last two centuries. Unlike the description of schizophrenia, which has evolved but is essentially unchanged since the inception of psychiatry, sexual behaviors and experiences have been seen in a variety of ways, and what constitutes a disorder or a condition has changed radically. Catalogs of sexual behaviors and the putative causes for them have long existed in medicine, and they have mostly been based on a sexual practice's degree of acceptability or its inability to be performed in a manner considered normal. In the HIV clinic, we have focused on the association of sexual behaviors with disruptions in functioning and the generation of distress or medical morbidity. In this section, we discuss three main topics: sexual behaviors that have become addictions, those conditions where patients have diminished sexual functions, and those conditions where patients are disturbed by the disruption of traditional sexual functioning.

Paraphilias

We define paraphilias as disorders of motivated behavior involving sex that are similar in pattern and nature to addictions. They are characterized by a craving for and a consuming interest in a particular type of sexual activity that is out of control and that displaces interest in other activities. This craving interferes with normal relationship development. The term can be broken into the components *para* (next to) and *philia* (love), which emphasize that the person is attracted to the object of his or her sexual desire in a way that is related to love but not the same as love. The central themes that tie the assorted paraphilic behaviors together are the addictive quality and the disorder that emerge from the pursuit of the behavior.

Paraphilias have been a controversial subject in psychiatry. This is in part because of the social, political, and religious ramifications of sexual behavior, as well as the strongly held views about acceptable and unacceptable sexual activity. At various times, society has defined homosexuality and many other behaviors as paraphilic without a clear distinction between illegal or unacceptable sexual behavior and the concept of sexual disorders as clinical entities. Does the desire for a sexual behavior that is unacceptable constitute a disorder? The desire for extramarital sexual behavior can cause many problems but hardly seems in the same category as the driven person who expends enormous resources and sacrifices all of his relationships in the pursuit of anonymous contacts with prostitutes. Defining paraphilia has the same problem as defining addiction described in the previous chapter. Many behaviors have the capacity to produce addictions but occur in normal life. They become paraphilic as they get out of control. They follow in much the same cycle as described in Chapter 5 (refer to Fig. 5.3).

Historically, the effort to define paraphilia has often focused on the degree of abnormality of the behavior. The presumption here is that even an interest in particular behaviors defines the person as having a disorder. Other definitions focus on the potential for injury to another person and make paraphilia a condition in which one of the parties either does not or cannot consent. This might suggest that a person has a disorder if he or she has sexual interaction with a partner who is under the legal age, whereas another person whose only sexual outlet is addiction to sex with a particular type of inanimate object does not have a disorder. We find it more useful to emphasize that the behavior causes problems or interferes with other activities. Some patients present with sexual addictions to "normal" sexual behaviors and have these relationships in a consensual manner, but they are nonetheless disordered and have a paraphilia.

Essentially, paraphilia is sexual behavior that disorders life rather than enriches it. When the behavioral cycle begins to get out of control, most people are able to restrain their behavior, but patients with paraphilia develop intense cravings for particular behaviors and continue the behavior even after it gets out of control. Over time, the particular behavior that they crave becomes more "stereotypical," meaning that it becomes more and more the same and focused on specific repeated activity. It also becomes more important that the sexual object remain the same as much as possible. Setting, time, manner of initiation, location, and other elements such as being intoxicated or wearing certain clothes may also become stereotyped.

Although there is no such thing as a typical paraphilia, most patients describe initial exposure to a particular sexual behavior that was overwhelmingly emotionally charged. In patients with sexual paraphilias directed at children, often their own sexual initiation took place in settings that were coercive or traumatic.

In the case of patients with exhibitionism and voyeurism, often an accidental exposure occurred that was very exciting or even terrifying. Following this, there is often a strong craving for the behavior. Patients may resist the behavior for years, but often at some critical juncture their resistance is overwhelmed and they begin a pattern of increasing pursuit of the behavior, sometimes gradually at first, and then ultimately they become consumed by it.

Paraphilic sex may or may not involve another person. Some paraphilias involve an addiction to collecting, touching, or possessing certain objects that have a sexual connotation for the patient. They may be addicted to sex that involves specialized devices or instruments, such as enemas or autoerotic asphyxiation, or they may be addicted to nonhuman partners, known as zoophilia. Some patients require injury or self-injury as part of the activity, and the sexual behavior may take on a bizarre ritualized form. The sexual behaviors of zoophilia or necrophilia are sufficiently beyond the capacity of most people to understand that many see them as fundamentally different than "ordinary" paraphilic behaviors, suggesting a different pathology or a necessary comorbidity.

Paraphilias also do not necessarily require that the patient experience an orgasm at the time of the event. Some patients are addicted to nonconsummatory behaviors, such as exhibitionism, frotteurism, and sadomasochism. In these behaviors the sexual release may occur at the time of the behavior or may occur later with masturbation.

Many people engage in behaviors that might be considered paraphilic, just as many people use intoxicants such as alcohol. Like the effects of alcohol and other reinforcing intoxicants on social interactions, used in moderation they may add spice to one's sexual life. Many of the behaviors that can develop into a paraphilia are not abnormal in themselves and are positive rather than negative for most people who engage in them. However, unlike the data with substance abuse, where use-to-abuse ratios have been studied to some extent, little is known about paraphilic behavior outside of disorders. Some behaviors seem to have a high degree of addictiveness and are almost always associated with the development of a disorder. Also, like substance abuse, some patients are addicted from their first exposure to a behavior and are out of control almost immediately, whereas others have a long experience with a behavior that gradually gets out of control. Other behaviors clearly have a paraphilic quality to them, but add a pleasurable dimension to sexuality and may never get out of control.

The most legally proscribed of sexual behaviors are those that involve nonconsensual sex or injure another person, such as paraphilic rape or pedophilia. Patients are aware of the illegality of the behavior and rationalize their behavior, but they are also driven by it and are unable to substitute other behaviors. Here the addictive quality is most obvious, as some people will commit suicide over their cravings, whereas others will lose all sense of control over their desires and commit certain acts with the direct purpose of being caught so as to escape the throes of their drive.

Other behaviors are less obviously harmful to others but are equally out of control. A common example is exhibitionism, which is often described by patients as irresistible. This is often seen as a nuisance crime, so that patients may have been caught on numerous occasions but had few consequences. Despite this, they may suddenly find themselves facing or having had serious consequences. Even those who face these consequences may expose themselves in settings where they are certain to be caught and then describe their urges as irresistible.

Knowledge and data must temper attitudes toward potentially addictive behaviors. Some behaviors are intensely addictive and have unacceptably high risks compared to the positive contribution they produce. Other behaviors produce disorders only in a modest subset of practitioners while enriching the lives of others. The role for health care providers is to recognize a disorder early and then intervene effectively. Issues of judgment are always difficult to discuss, but behaviors that lead to injury, risk, and impairments in functioning must be discussed with patients and considered as potential disorders.

The diagnosis of paraphilia is often difficult, as patients may be very reluctant to discuss the behavior with anyone. The screening questions are straightforward and should be asked by all clinicians as part of the standard sexual history. Patients are often relieved as the diagnosis is made, and they discover that they are not the only one with the problem and that they can get help.

The description of paraphilia is germane to this book because some patients are addicted to behaviors with a high risk of HIV and other health problems. Paraphilias are frequently highly repetitive and often become out of the patient's control. The drive to engage in the behavior is similar to that described by other addicted patients in Chapter 5. Patients are often aware of the self-destructive nature of their practice, but their intrusive cravings interfere with their better judgment. Although they are often in denial at first presentation, they describe an irresistible urge, a sense of physical craving, an appetite, or a hungry state that makes the behavior difficult or impossible to stop.

Data from research in this area are quite scarce for HIV issues. Although a few studies of criminal sex offenders have found no increase in HIV infection,[1] the best data in the area come from studies of men who dress as women and work as prostitutes. It is clear that the rates of high risk associated with this behavior are very high. The numbers of partners each year are often in excess of 1,500, with high rates of unsafe sexual practices and high rates of sexually transmitted diseases. The HIV rates are dependent on the geographic region studied, and studies are quite scarce. Additionally, most of the studies on HIV risk behavior in these populations identify patients by their actions, and few studies have been done to ascertain the degree to which the behavior is motivated by paraphilia. Despite these criticisms, these studies may be interpreted to suggest that men with this paraphilia have high rates of both HIV and risky behavior.[2-7]

Paraphilias that involve frequent sexual contact with anonymous partners increase the risk for HIV and other sexually transmitted diseases. These patients may have in excess of hundreds of contacts each year. The driven quality of the behavior makes it hard for patients to use safer sexual practices, and the intensity of the drive may lead patients to disregard ordinary precautions in the heat of the moment. Other risks include serious injuries from assaults involving premature or unwanted sexual advances, as well as the serious injuries frequently seen in patients with violent and physical paraphilias. Some patients actually describe an excitement associated with risk and may find the risk of becoming infected with HIV adds to the paraphilic drive.

Both heterosexual and homosexual men can develop paraphilias, which can lead to the rapid spread of HIV. Prostitution is a vector for transmission, and patients addicted to visiting prostitutes may consume enormous resources pursuing their addictive behavior. Heterosexual men may have large numbers of partners, spend almost all of their time in pursuit of sexual activity, and have their behavior disorder their social, occupational, and romantic lives. Paraphilia leads away from sustained, intimate, and growth-producing relationships and interferes with the important developments that a commitment to something beyond one's appetite can bring. In this way, it resembles other addictions.

Homosexuality and Paraphilia

If the hallmarks of paraphilia are the lack of sustained, intimate relationships, the lack of the ability to function in other areas (such as social and occupational functions), and the development of an increasing disorder over time, it is difficult to equate homosexual behavior with paraphilia. At one time, psychiatry identified homosexuality as a paraphilia. The evidence to support this view was that homosexuality was an abnormal behavior. Our experience in working with gay patients does not support the view that all homosexual behavior leads to paraphilia, and we have seen many sustained, intimate, and growth-directed homosexual relationships.

The ideas that surround homosexuality emerge from culture, manners, morality, and traditions, as well as natural drives and human nature. As clinicians, we direct our attention toward medical and health issues. This means that the popular perception that homosexual men are unable to sustain a long-term relationship and are always promiscuous must be confronted by clinicians in helping patients to redirect their efforts toward better health.

Although the research is poor, there may well be an increased risk for the development of paraphilia in men who have sex with men. Paraphilic disorders, as we have described them, are vastly more common in men than in women. Women have a variety of sexual disorders, but appetitive addictions to increasingly stereotyped sexual or parasexual behaviors appear to be rare in women. In part, this protects heterosexual men, as their female partners are less willing to tolerate the stereotypical addictive sexual behaviors than are male partners. Little quality research has been done on the true epidemiology of paraphilias among gay men, but it is a significant clinical problem found in our work. A clinician should screen for and consider the diagnosis when patients present with a pattern of disorders that are otherwise difficult to explain.

It is also worthwhile to mention that paraphilias emerge from behavior, just as other addictions. The same comorbid risks we described for substance abuse in Chapter 5 have an influence on sexual behavior and risk. Depression may bring about a dissatisfaction with usual sexual activity and lead to sexual extremes that may be addictive. Being intoxicated may lead to unsafe, exciting, and addictive sexual practices. Extraversion may lead to trying things that introverts would be averse to exploring. Introversion may be a barrier to finding partners and may lead to addictive forms of autoeroticism and anonymous sexual interactions. Thus, in considering the risk of developing paraphilia, it is important for the clinician to know the patient as well as the behavior. In treating paraphilia, much as in addictions to other behaviors, the comorbid condition must also be treated.

Treating Paraphilia

When patients describe a worsening syndrome of intrusive, driven sexual behavior that is affecting their lives and seems addictive in quality, treatment is similar to that described in Chapter 5. Although overly simplified, we have outlined the steps of treatment. They may occur simultaneously but have differing goals and strategies. The steps of treatment are as follows:

1. Induction of the patient role
2. Detoxification
3. Treatment of comorbid conditions
4. Rehabilitation
5. Maintenance and prevention of relapse

Induction

In the induction phase, the goal is to induce the patient to accept the need for a rehabilitation-directed treatment plan. Few patients arrive having decided they will completely give up the behavior that has come to dominate their life, or that they are willing to make the sacrifices necessary to achieve this goal. They are often brought by partners or family members, occasionally by bosses or other supervisors, and even by referring doctors. They also come under duress as directed by courts and law enforcement agencies or employee assistance programs.

In the initial interview, the focus is on establishing the diagnosis. We then describe the condition, the treatment goals, and the treatment plan. Patients often reject the diagnosis, deny that they have any problem, or tell clinicians that this is a behavior they cannot change or control. An important element of this part of the treatment is to convert the patient from the goal of relief from consequences, their usual initial goal, to a goal of improving function.

This involves three simultaneous processes. The first is confrontation, which includes a clear description of the trouble the patient is in, the phenomenology of paraphilia, and comparisons with alcohol and other addictions. We find that confrontation works best with a smile and a warm approach, rather than presenting hard facts in an accusatory way, such as is popularly seen on television shows and called "an intervention." Patients often vigorously deny their problem, but we smile at their objections and rationalizations. We gently point out that they are in trouble and need help. Part of this process is emphasizing that the behavior must stop, is out of control, and is ruining the person's life.

The second part of induction is the presentation of an alternative life picture. We present hope for a life that is better, richer, and more fun. Most patients have not contemplated a life without their behaviors, and their paraphilias may be the central focus of their lives. Most often, patients present a goal of freedom to pursue their behaviors without consequences. To persuade a patient to consider an alternative life raises both hope and conflict within the patient. We have found that a useful suggestion at this point is to encourage the patient to try a year without the behavior, and if life is not better, to go back to his or her previous way of life. This can sometimes bypass the endless negotiations about cutting down and trying to do it less that may confound this part of treatment.

The third part of induction is literally to describe the role of the patient. We emphasize the term *rehabilitation* and make comparisons with physical rehabilitation after a stroke. This emphasizes that it will not be easy or comfortable to change, but it also stresses the sense of relearning something and getting back to health. We point out that in this sort of problem, the patient has to do most of the work. Patients with problem behaviors often get overvalued ideas about being cured by pills or some intense therapeutic insight. They may wish to discuss why they do it for years and never get to how to stop doing it. Ultimately, success depends on getting the patient to commit to treatment.

At some point in treatment, a pharmacologic drive reduction with drugs that decrease one's drives by altering the androgen/testosterone axis can be offered to patients. Studies have shown that antiandrogens, estrogens, medroxyprogesterone, and, most recently, gonadotropin-releasing agents (GN-RH) such as leuprolide (Lupron) and its slow release form can all decrease sexual drive. Some studies suggest that the paraphilic drive is diminished less than the drive for normal sexual activity.[8] All the drugs have significant side effects and toxicities. Consultation with an expert should be obtained before using these agents.

The degree of benefit from these drugs is patient-specific and quite variable. Some patients describe complete relief from cravings for behaviors they identify as abnormal with no effect on the ones they consider normal. Cravings for anonymous sex, painful or destructive behaviors, and high-frequency, high-risk encounters may diminish, or even completely disappear, without affecting the ability to enjoy sex within relationships. On the other hand, some patients describe a general reduction of their sex drive with a commensurate reduction in drives for paraphilic behaviors.

The decision to use pharmacologic measures is made on a case-by-case basis. We usually mention it in the induction phase but may not recommend it until later, if at all. We have not found pharmacotherapy to be the primary treatment; it is adjunctive to the other treatments. Patients who cannot control their behavior, fail other interventions, or simply want their behavior to be easier to resist find pharmacotherapy to be a useful consideration.

Several choices are available, but we have had the most experience with Depo-Provera, oral Provera, and Depot-leuprolide (Lupron). Other clinicians support the usage of many other drugs, including selective serotonin reuptake inhibitor (SSRI) antidepressants, Buspirone, and neuroleptics. None of them has been approved for treating paraphilia, however, with only modest data documenting their usage.

Oral Provera is inexpensive and often effective. The oral dose for men is given daily, and it has significant side effects. Depo-Provera can be given by injection on a weekly to monthly basis. It is also relatively inexpensive and has many side effects. In our experience, Depot-leuprolide is the best tolerated, most expensive, and easiest to use. Since the FDA does not approve it for this use, reimbursement from insurance companies is quite problematic.

Detoxification

As in all addictive behaviors, treatment cannot proceed while the patient is in the throes of the addiction. The purpose of the detoxification step is to stop the behavior. This sometimes requires an admission to the hospital, and patients often do not wish to be admitted to a psychiatry floor for a diagnosis of paraphilia. This is a reasonable stance to take, given the way medical records are reviewed by insurance companies, hospital reviewers, and a host of other administrative parties. Few patients are thrilled to have their insurance company know the intimate details of their sexual life, and many people see the word *pervert* when they read the word *paraphilia*. Some patients present with suicidal feelings associated with their behaviors, and their level of desperation makes hospitalization easier for them to accept and less stigmatizing. This also allows the rationale for hospital admission to be more acceptable to reviewers and family members, and the documentation can focus on suicide issues even if the treatment focuses on the paraphila. With encouragement and support, most patients can stop their behaviors as outpatients.

If patients are not placed in immediate danger by their behaviors, outpatient treatment with frequent visits may be an acceptable alternative to inpatient care. Structured therapy is necessary, as described later, along with monitored activity. If patients are unable to stop their behaviors, we will likely intensify treatment with an inpatient or day hospital admission. Thus, the decision to move to a more aggressive treatment or restrictive setting is based on the risk to the patient, but it also considers the level of action on the patient's part to work toward cessation of the behavior. As described with substance use disorders, the key is to get the patient to do more if treatment is failing, not for the clinician to do more.

Treatment of Comorbid Conditions

The role of comorbid disorders is similar to that described for substance abuse in Chapter 5 and in the case example. They will not be reviewed exhaustively here, but depression, obsessive-compulsive disorder, substance use disorders, and personality must be assessed, because untreated disorders in these domains will almost certainly sabotage any treatment.

Rehabilitation

In the treatment of paraphilia, it is crucial for the patient to develop new patterns of behavior to replace the old ones. By the time most patients are diagnosed, their behavioral problems have reached significant levels. During patient evaluation, it is important to note the rigidity, stereotypicality and permanenceof the behavior, and the amount of time devoted to it. Few patients are willing to give up sexual activity altogether, and rehabilitation involves behavioral changes as much as cessation. In substance abuse, rehabilitation programs tell patients to change "people, places, and things." This philosophy stems from the Pavlovian idea that some of these things are triggers or associated stimuli that cue the behavior and help reinforce it, and that by eliminating or unlearning the associations, a patient will lessen his or her drive for the behavior.

Patients need to be committed to changing their lives and avoiding addictive behaviors. For this part of treatment, we find group therapy generally produces the best results. Certain topics regarding commitments can have a greater influence on a new patient when they come from fellow patients rather than from a clinician. These topics include confrontation, strategies for preventing relapse, ways of coping with cravings (an inevitable part of recovery), and accepting the idea that the behavior is pathological and represents a disorder (often the term *disease* is used). Twelve-step programs based on the Alcoholics Anonymous (AA) method are very useful and may actually function as the backbone of treatment. Groups can also be developed around a variety of relapse prevention models. Patients may attend groups run by local experts but remain in the care of the HIV clinical team. "Sexaholics Anonymous" groups have been established in most cities, and referral networks can help patients find the right group to join.

In some settings, group treatments are unavailable and some patients are unwilling to participate in them or do not find them helpful. Individual therapy can also be successful, and several models of treatment have been proposed, including relapse prevention-based models as well as a variety of other behavioral approaches. We find it useful to be willing to try different treatments if one approach fails. This does not mean that the patient alone can direct the treatment, since all behavioral disorders seek ways to reassert themselves. We will even agree to a plan we think will not succeed if it poses little risk, provided the patient will agree to a more aggressive plan in the case of failure.

Successful rehabilitation requires that patients fill up their lives with new behaviors to help the old ones dissipate. Some appetite for the old behaviors is always present, and as rehabilitation proceeds one must be careful to avoid reintroducing behavioral temptations. Patients with pedophilia, for example, cannot work in daycare centers, even with daily groups and an ocean of Lupron. Patients with paraphilias that involve impulsive anonymous sex partners need to avoid intoxication even if they have no alcohol problems, and they also need to avoid the kinds of places where opportunities abound. For any of this to work, the patient must decide that he or she needs help and wants to change. Sexual behaviors have intrinsic biologic drives associated with them, and they feel normal even when they are destructive. Patients cannot be forced to want a different type of sexual attraction or feeling, but they can change their behavior and, by doing so, they can be free of the tyranny of sexual disorders that control their lives.

Maintenance

The most difficult aspect of addictions is that they can reemerge at any time. The cycle of motivated behavior, once kindled, seems to be present and waiting even years later. Patients may relapse early or late and often feel sad or angry that they have worked so hard and so long to fight their disorder, only to relapse at a critical moment. Maintenance involves the avoidance of conditioned stimuli, such as people, places, and things that will provoke the behavior. It requires vigilance about patterns of behavior that lead to relapse. It also involves an ongoing commitment to treatment. We recommend targeted groups or individual therapy, but several of our patients continue to control their paraphilia by attending AA meetings to maintain abstinence.

Sexual Disorders Other than Paraphilias

Sexual and Gender Identity

A confusing array of terminology has developed in the arena of sexuality. We will use the term *sex* to describe the biologically determined set of sexual organs a person is born with, and to describe the behaviors of sexual expression. Disorders in this domain are rare, but sometimes patients born with chromosomes that determine male sex have ambiguous or female genitalia, and vice versa. Some chromosomal abnormalities include extra or deleted sex chromosomes. In large part, we will not discuss chromosomal disorders or ambiguous genitalia here. We will use the term *sexual partner preference* to describe the choice of partner a person prefers. The term *gender identity* will describe the role the patient has chosen.

Some men like to wear clothing that is typically worn by women, and they do so for many reasons. The term *transvestite* simply describes the behavior of wearing female apparel, but it has traditionally implied that the clothes are worn for the sake of erotic stimulation. This behavior can lead to paraphilia, and patients may become addicted to sexual activities that involve wearing particular clothes. Some men and women also choose to cross-dress for other reasons. They may enjoy the attention they receive during the behavior or they may wish to express their attraction to a particular type of role and identity.

The terms *transsexual* and *transgender* are used to describe those with the urge to become members of the opposite sex or who identify themselves as such. Their gender identity, the sense of being male or female, may be distorted by their desire to be the opposite sex or the dislike of their own sex. The term *gender dysphoria* suggests a dissatisfaction with one's biologically determined sexual nature. Some patients see themselves as transgendered and have a strong sense of gender identity, albeit with their opposite gender. Since gender identity does not determine the sex of the preferred partner, patients who are biologically male but feel they should be female may prefer male or female partners.

Patients with an altered gender identity, or the desire to change sexual identity, have been traditionally described as disordered because of this desire or feeling. We do not agree that this is uniformly the case, but agree that many patients are suffering. Several studies of these patients have shown high rates of other psychiatric conditions.[9] When dealing with these sexual issues, the primary issues facing a clinician are whether the patient with HIV also has a disorder, and how to identify the nature of the disorder. The term *disorder* implies that the patient is unable to perform some function in such a way that prevents him or her from having a complete life. Some of the judgment is subjective, but in other cases it is quite clear. Sexual identity beliefs that lead to behaviors often are the most problematic when patients have other significant vulnerabilities, such as problems of disposition and personality. These problems can be intimately linked with personality and are hard to diagnose and treat as separate conditions.

During the interview with a patient, we focus on function, quality of life, and longevity, and we discuss with patients whether matters of sexuality adversely affect these areas. If so, they may require treatment. Expert care is often required for this arena, but to persuade patients to go for treatment, clinicians must understand the issues, including high risk behavior for HIV and STD transmission, adherence to treatment, risk of physical injury and irresponsible surgical alteration, and impairments of social, occupational, and romantic functions. It cannot be emphasized too strongly that patients with transgender issues may not in fact be disordered by the sexual issue, but may be suffering from a comorbid psychiatric condition that is easily overlooked if the focus is on sex alone. Therefore, the expert evaluation should include a wider search for psychiatric disorders that occur much more commonly, including affective disorders, substance use disorders, personality disorders, and life story disorders (for a discussion of life story disorders, see Chapter 7). As a last issue, we live in a culture that has developed a strong commitment to the primacy of feelings and emotional life over promises, rules, social obligations, and other inconvenient behavioral constraints. Many of the patients with identity difficulties see themselves as victims rather than authors of their misadventures in life to the point where they are unable to make progress or resist self-destruction. We have seen many patients who wish to solve the problems of their lives with interventions directed solely at their feelings without regard to their function. Cosmetic surgery, cosmetic medication, or cosmetic psychotherapy designed to make patients feel better without improving their functioning often pose significant risks that vulnerable patients may be unable or unwilling to appreciate. Often these interventions do not increase functioning, quality of life, or longevity, and all of them have significant risks. Sex reassignment surgery is an aggressive treatment for a problem that may not be solved after the operation. Retrospective reviews of patients who have undergone such an operation demonstrate that many are no happier, no more functional, and no less impaired after their treatment. Once the surgery has been completed, the changes cannot be undone, and efforts to reverse the surgery often cause more problems than they cure.

The job of medical care providers is to carefully evaluate the nature of problems and advocate for treatments that have a desirable ratio of benefit to risk. This often means that sex-reassignment surgery may not be the best approach to solving a problem in a patient's life, despite his or her absolute commitment to the treatment. This is a difficult conversation to have with patients who come to the physician having already decided that this treatment will solve all their problems. Similar problems arise regularly in psychiatry and medicine. The most obvious case is the patient who requests an amputation because of the delusion that parasites are infesting his arm. Less clear is the woman with anorexia nervosa who wants breast augmentation so her parents will stop complaining about how thin she has become, or who wishes to be an exotic dancer or star in pornographic movies. Should the clinician deliver the treatment to any patient with the money, or does the provider have an obligation to advise against or even to refuse an intervention he or she sees as potentially having more risk than benefit? Certainly, the limited data on the outcomes of various sexual reassignment procedures give us pause about recommending the practice. Although better data on more selected patients may change this stance, at this moment we need more critical thought, less politics, and more self-restraint.

Sexual Dysfunction

This section focuses on the diminished ability to have or enjoy sexual activity. The literature in this area is extensive for patients not affected by HIV. There has been an explosion of interest in the sexual functions of chronically medically ill patients in the last 20 years, as clinicians have realized the degree to which medical conditions, medications, injuries, and physical deconditioning can aversely affect sexual functioning. The idea that sexual activity is for the young and healthy has given way to a general clinical interest in sexual issues of the elderly and to a lesser extent those with chronic medical problems.

HIV is a condition that may impair sexual functioning because of any resulting medical illnesses, debilitation, or other health-related issues. Problems in sexual functioning may also result from anxiety about chronic HIV infection, general medication side effects, opportunistic infections, and damage to the nervous system caused by HIV. In addition, medications for HIV that cause neuropathy may have a direct effect on sexual functioning. Treatments for HIV may also lead to diabetes, which can result in sexual dysfunction by causing neuropathy, chronic illness, body habitus alteration, and even dehydration and hypovolemia. As with all medical problems, the complaint of sexual dysfunction should generate a differential diagnosis. Although the literature on sexual dysfunction in patients with HIV is scarce, it is clear that the difficulties in sexual function are most often multifactorial, and perseverance is required to effect improvements in this domain.

Although many authors divide sexual functioning into desire, arousal, and orgasm phases, many patients have problems at more than one phase. Also, an erectile dysfunction may cause diminished desire and anxiety, leading to impaired orgasm. Similarly for women, a lack of lubrication may lead to pain with intercourse, avoidance of sexual activity, and a loss of the ability to experience orgasm. It is worthwhile to try to get patients to describe the exact nature of their difficulty, as this can lead to a more coherent treatment plan.

HIV-infected patients may experience dysfunction in any of these phases caused by HIV's consequences and medical treatments. The type and cause of the sexual dysfunction determine the correct treatment. It is difficult to get patients to talk about the problems they encounter, yet this is essential for allowing the clinician to develop clear ideas about the potential causes of dysfunction. Problems range from neuropathy to distortion of body image, and causes range from medications, consequences of viral injury or associated opportunistic infections, to psychological injuries from body changes because of lipodystrophy.

Many HIV-infected patients lose their sexual appetite or desire. They feel uninterested in sexual activity or have specific impairments in sexual functions. For men with advanced disease, a loss of libido may be a harbinger of some more ominous medical problem or simply a matter of decreased stamina and energy. Some patients have been found to have low testosterone levels and benefit from testosterone supplementation or replacement.[9] Other patients experience the restoration of their libido with time and antiviral therapy. It is often a partner that brings the problem to clinical attention, but most patients will note a decreased interest in sex if directly asked.

Erectile dysfunction, arousal failure, and the resultant frustration can actually be easier to treat than problems regarding sexual interest. Neuropathy, medications, systemic illness, and intoxication are common causes of erectile dysfunction, and they can also interfere with sensation in women. It is essential to evaluate the patient for medical causes, but problems can often be resolved with continued treatment. Sildenafil (Viagra), tadalafil (Cialis), vardenafil (Levitra), mechanical intervention, and other therapies are available, but these may be intimidating for patients. Consultation from a team that uses both mechanical and psychological strategies may be useful in some cases.

Anorgasmia, altered ejaculation, and other orgasmic dysfunctions can be very disturbing for patients. Again, the evaluation of changes in a patient's medical condition and medication is critical. Many patients benefit from evaluation and treatment, which usually involves consultation from a specialty clinic or practice.

As mentioned earlier, many drugs can cause a decreased interest in sexual activity or affect arousal, lubrication, and orgasm. It is also a common problem for patients to notice their sexual dysfunction and blame the medication they're taking for the problem. This can affect compliance with medications and the relationship with health care providers. Reassurance that the effects are likely to diminish with time and that antiretrovirals may actually improve sexual functioning over time is very important. It is also crucial to involve the patient's sexual partner in this discussion. Questions about the necessity of the treatment or about ameliorating the sacrifices associated with the treatment can be addressed when both parties can help make the decision.

Decreased sexual interest and sexual dysfunction can be caused by the physical problems associated with HIV, but they can also be caused by the patients' subjective sense of their attractiveness, wellness, and psychological views of the future. These problems, however, can be rectified in individual or couples therapy. When no other cause can be determined, it is reasonable to try an empiric intervention using medications such as sildenafil (Viagra), vardenafil (Levitra) or tadalafil (Cialis). Testosterone treatments have also become something of a fad for HIV patients, yet they have been effective in improving the sexual functions, moods, and satisfaction of patients with diminished testosterone levels.[9]

Depression should be considered a factor for any patient with decreased sexual drive or activity. Depression can affect all phases of sexual functioning, and some of the medications used in treating HIV or the commonly co-occurring hepatitis C cause depression (most notably efavirenz and interferon alpha). Additionally, HIV-infected patients have high rates of depression to begin with, and patients with depression often present with complaints about sexual interest or functioning.

Many of the antidepressants have sexual side effects as well, complicating this problem. Selective serotonin reuptake inhibitors (SSRIs) may cause anorgasmia, delayed ejaculation, and decreased libido. In our experience, they rarely cause erectile difficulty but may do so because of decreased interest. They can sometimes be useful when a patient complains of premature ejaculation. Tricyclic antidepressants block both alpha receptors and muscarinic receptors, and can cause difficulties with erection, ejaculation, and vaginal dryness. Although these problems tend to attenuate with time, they improve more slowly in sicker patients. Atypical agents such as mirtazapine and nefazodone also block these receptors but to a lesser extent, and they may still have a negative effect on sexual functioning in particular patients. Tricyclic and heterocyclic agents seem to have less effect on libido than SSRI drugs and therefore may produce the paradoxical effect of a patient who finally has the will, but not the way. It is also important to note sexual problems before initiating treatment with antidepressants or antiretrovirals so that, as patients improve, they do not discontinue the very treatments most likely to restore sexual functions. In the end, an effective diagnosis of depression and proper treatment often lead to improvements in sexual function, a better treatment outcome, and compliance as well.

A final issue is that of sexual dysfunction in the context of relationship problems. Couples' problems for gay men are undertreated and underdiagnosed. Couples may need long-term relationship therapy, and they may need the suggestion to come from their medical providers. Most places have skilled therapists who can help gay couples improve their quality of life and can address issues of intimacy, sexual functioning, and relationship problems that affect the couple's sexual functioning.

Case: A Couple

F is a 42-year-old Hispanic physician who was born outside the United States and has practiced medicine for many years in the eastern United States. He was referred from another city for evaluation of relationship problems and non-compliance with HIV medications. His long-time partner, G, accompanied him for his evaluation and for most of the treatment visits.

F was born to an upper middle-class family and had no childhood difficulties. His family history was strongly positive for heart disease, and one maternal aunt had been depressed and drank alcohol to excess. His mother and many members of her family had experienced postpartum blues, with the result that F and his two sisters had stayed with his father's sister for a month or two after their births; all had been raised on formula rather than breast milk.

He became sexually active in his teens and had several girlfriends until around the age of 18. He said these relationships were okay, but throughout high school he was attracted to a male teacher who was gay. He began a sexual relationship with this teacher just before graduation and continued to see him for two years before the relationship ended. F attended medical school and kept his sexual orientation a secret from his family. He stated that, although his mother always knew, he felt his father "couldn't handle it." His family supported his decision to move to the United States, and he made yearly visits home. He later informed his parents of his relationship with his current partner, G, whom they liked and accepted, but they were unaware of his HIV status.

F completed residency training at a prestigious academic center. He was financially and academically successful. He never married, had no children, and mostly had male romantic partners since coming to the United States. At the time of presentation, he had been in a stable relationship with G for five years. He had no other active medical problems, was taking no medication, and had no known drug allergies. He was diagnosed with an HIV infection six years before our evaluation, and by the time of the evaluation he had a CD4 cell count of 500 cells/mm^3 and a viral load of 35,000. He had begun therapy at a CD4 cell count of 280 cells/mm^3. He had been treated with a triple therapy regimen of nelfinavir and AZT/3TC (as Combivir), but had stopped taking his medications six months before his evaluation. He had been treated several times for sexually transmitted diseases, including genital herpes, gonorrhea, and syphilis. He had additionally undergone empiric treatment for prostatitis on at least three occasions.

F had a history of occasional alcohol excess that included binges when he would drink to the point of intoxication each night for a couple of months at a time. He always stopped this behavior, however, before things got out of control. He never used illicit drugs but had self-prescribed sleep medications, including several different benzodiazepines.

F had previously met with a psychologist and a psychiatrist. He had seen the psychologist when he was much younger in an effort to change his sexual orientation to heterosexual, but confessed he had little hope this would occur. Thus, his therapy with the psychologist lasted for only two sessions. He consulted the psychiatrist after his last romantic breakup. He said the treatment had focused mostly on discussing his sexual fantasies, which consisted of sex with partners he described as "sleazy young men." F said that he and his psychiatrist came to interpret these men as symbolizing an anxiety about castration, and that his psychiatrist had told him his homosexuality resulted from his fear of castration by his father for his intense connection with his mother. The interpretation went on to explain that by trying to sexually please "symbolic father surrogates" he was trying to prevent his own castration, and by trying to sexually please young, sleazy men he was trying to please his mother sexually, but had to substitute men for women to avoid the anger of his father.

F's physician referred him to us when he abruptly stopped taking his antivirals and decided to take a drug holiday. G was very upset by F's decision to stop taking his HIV medication. G had an undetectable viral load on the same drug combination and was extremely conscientious about his medication. Both had the same physician, who met with them to discuss F's decision to stop medication and discovered conflict between the partners concerning this stop, as well as several other issues. G believed that F intended to break up and that F had exhibited the same pattern when he had ended his last long-term relationship, also of five years' duration. The relationship had been with a person well known to G.

During his private evaluation, F described a pattern of relationships characterized by intense love for a partner, usually a couple of years younger than him, that would last three to five years. He said during this time he would be satisfied with the relationship and feel he had finally met the right person. He would then begin fighting with his partner, becoming irritable over what he called "stupid things." He would also find fault with his partner, find him less attractive, and begin to notice other younger men. Eventually, he would break off each relationship and go on a spree of anonymous sexual encounters with younger men, even with several partners at a time. He would always loathe himself after these events and promise himself not to engage in such behavior again. He said he would scold himself in his mother's voice, calling himself a fag, a whore, or a slut in Spanish, and imagine how disgusted his father would be with his behavior.

During these times F would have difficulty sleeping, stay up much of the night, and eventually go out looking for sexual partners. He said when he tried to resist the thoughts of what he wanted, it became impossible to concentrate on work, and he had actually left his work to have brief trysts. He was convinced that this was how he had been infected with HIV, as he had acquired all of his sexually transmitted diseases (STDs) during these periods. He described an intense feeling of self-loathing permeating these times, missing his previous partner, remembering all of the good things, and feeling he had betrayed the only person he could ever love. He described how alcohol played a part in these periods.

F also said that at these times he would lament being homosexual. He would think about how he had disappointed his father, how he could have been married and loved only women, and how he had betrayed his family. These thoughts were accompanied by both suicidal thoughts and fantasies of self-castration, as he would fantasize that, if he were castrated, he could resist his impulses.

His description of his sexual behavior with his long-term partners was different than during his promiscuous episodes. With his partners, sex was more loving and mutual, whereas in the promiscuous phases it was degrading and humiliating. He had intense fantasies of degradation during sex with anonymous partners and had actually been hurt on a couple of occasions. He would permit anything and preferred abusive, rough sexual encounters. He also preferred a different type of partner. His relationships were with bright men who were successful and well groomed. For his anonymous partners, he preferred slightly tough and dirty-looking men, in their teens to early twenties, and often with drug problems.

F stated that in G he had found his soul mate. G was a successful administrator, well liked, smart, and good company. F had been completely in love with him until about six months ago, when he began to find him impossibly irritating and fussy. He initially decided that G had changed, but then realized after discussion with his friends that it was his own problem. He reported he had continued the relationship with G despite increased cravings for his old patterns of behavior. He had stopped having sex with G about two months before the evaluation and had had two sexual sprees, each lasting one day. G knew of these affairs, and this was part of why he had insisted that F come for evaluation.

In addition, G would not allow F to drink because of an incident three years before in which F had been drinking to excess and had a public fight. At the time, F was taking alprazolam in ever-increasing doses to sleep. About a month before his evaluation, he had been warned about self-prescribing by a pharmacist, and his doctor refused to give him alprazolam unless he underwent an evaluation. He decided to stop it on his own but admitted he had not slept well in more than a month without it. On several occasions he had obtained alprazolam again when he felt desperate that he could not sleep.

The private meeting with G added little new information. G was a high-functioning 34-year-old white male. He was carefully dressed, soft spoken, and elegant. He had had an unremarkable childhood and family history, except for a vague report of nervous breakdowns in remote family members. His family had suspected he was gay in high school and accepted it. He had gone to college and completed an MBA, had continued to have close ties with his mother, and had many friends. He was active in his community, had been involved exclusively with men, and had no medical problems outside of his HIV. G believed he had been infected in one of his two other long-term relationships, both of which had been with HIV-infected men, and he admitted he had not been careful enough. He had received yearly testing and started treatment just before meeting F. G had more than 1,000 CD4 cells/mm^3 and an undetectable viral load, and he was religious about taking his medication.

G had met F through a friend who had been in a long-term relationship with F. He thought F was struggling with the "South American macho thing" about being gay and hurting his family, but that he needed to get over it. He also thought that F exaggerated his problem so he could go on one of his self-destructive "boy benders" and "alcohol benders." He described F as spoiled and self-indulgent, but also wonderful and brilliant. He said that although he was committed to trying to make things work, they had to get better or he was going to move on. He denied any relationships outside his involvement with F and said that he did not cheat. He said he knew F had cheated because he had stopped having sex and that F was "too spoiled to go without sex."

The topics of discussion for the session with both F and G were depression and paraphilia. F agreed enthusiastically about the diagnosis of depression but seemed reluctant about the paraphilia. He felt his depression explained everything adequately, and G was able to describe many other symptoms that lent credibility to depression as a diagnosis. G was concerned about the diagnosis of paraphilia but believed that F could stop his behaviors if he were treated because he had stopped his drinking and alprazolam abuse. A selective serotonin reuptake inhibitor (SSRI) antidepressant was discussed as a treatment option, both for its beneficial effect on treating depression and its potential to lessen sexual appetite and behaviors. F wanted to take a medication that was less likely to have sexual side effects, but ultimately he was persuaded to take sertraline and was titrated to a dose of 100 mg per day.

F came alone for follow-ups about every other week. At his fourth visit he admitted he was somewhat concerned about his sexual life. His mood was much better after six weeks of treatment, and his sleep had improved. He was more optimistic about the future and less self-deprecating, but he mentioned a continued longing for anonymous sex. He became more forthcoming about his preoccupation with sexual fantasies and the severity of his cravings. He admitted he had pressed G since the beginning of their relationship to engage in sexual behaviors that he found stimulating. Early in their relationship, F had experimented sexually with G, but G was unenthusiastic, and even when he was willing, it was not the same as the encounters with strangers had been. F was more forthcoming about the description of his sexual fantasies and admitted that he frequently fantasized during sex with G about other things. He had discussed an open relationship as well as group sex, both of which G refused to consider.

We discussed the issues of an intimate and therefore limited relationship with G, as opposed to the kind of relationship F had proposed. F admitted that he usually got whatever he wanted. He also said that his time with G, despite his perception that G was a fussy perfectionist with a narrow point of view, had been the best time of his life. He admitted that some part of him craved the excitement of the kind of sex life he would have if he broke up with G. Despite the inevitable self-loathing and excessive drinking, he was confident he would find someone new eventually, but he cried when he discussed giving up G.

F missed his next two appointments and then came with G about a month later. He was upset about having a paraphilia and admitted he was avoiding the issue. F described his strong drive for sex, which was intensified by alcohol intoxication. Leuprolide was presented as an option for sexual drive suppression, but with the renewed commitment to abstinence from alcohol that F and G had made, we decided not to use it and continued with psychotherapy and antidepressant medication alone. As his depression improved, F's ability to resist his impulses also seemed better. For the next year, F did well on his medications, he resumed antiviral treatment, and the relationship seemed stable. F persisted in thinking G was overreacting to his sexual drive, but he had no outside sexual contacts. He did resume occasional alcohol use, with many objections from G, but they continued to come to Baltimore once a month for sessions.

After a year of significant improvement, F had an incident involving too much alcohol and a public fight with G. In the aftermath, F agreed to attend Alcoholics Anonymous (AA) meetings once a week for a year to keep G from leaving. It was not until this point that F became committed to treatment and abstinence from both alcohol and outside sexual contact. His commitment to AA had a positive effect on the relationship with G and on other elements of his life. He continues to receive treatment for depression locally, and he sees me on rare occasions, usually with G. Both have undetectable viral loads and continue on medications.

Discussion

Although this case nicely demonstrates the straightforward approach of stopping a motivated behavior that had progressed to cause significant disorder and treating comorbid conditions, it also shows how a patient's conversion is crucial in the treatment of such addictive disorders. Any practitioner might recognize F's depression because the symptoms were distressing to him, yet he was enthusiastic about narrowing down a medical cause for his problems. The pattern of his sexual behavior was recognizable if directly discussed, but F downplayed the problematic nature of his rigid sexual appetites and strong drives. Because the behavior is gratifying in some way, it provides a reward to propagate the addictive cycle. Once involved in the addictive cycle, patients often have difficulty seeing the disorder that arises, a phenomenon now even colloquially referred to as denial. While the cycle was halted, F described very clearly how his sexual appetite was shaped over a series of experiences in which the more degrading the experience was, the more pleasure he derived from it.

In the diagram of addictive behavior (see Fig. 5.3), we can add several features. This is a positive feedback cycle: the more times it goes around, the more it spins out of control. Great effort must be made to stop the behavior early in the treatment, as the cycle is harder to stop the longer it continues. Also, the cycle has natural restraints in a normal life. Social factors; financial factors; work commitments; a partner, family, or friends; and an investment in one's future slow the cycle and control it. These factors predict that paraphilia develops, like other addictions, at transitions in life. Loss of one's job, partner, and financial stability, as well as geographic relocation with an attendant loss of social support, friends, and family, all favor the development of paraphilia. Young people making the transition from their family of origin to their adult role are vulnerable to a paraphilia disorder, and people in major transitions are more vulnerable than those in stable life circumstances.

F's paraphilia developed and worsened during episodes of depression and transition. It was important to identify factors that would slow his behavioral cycle. One of his stabilizing factors was his seemingly good relationship with G. His high socioeconomic status also proved to be a stabilizing factor, because he realized how deeply he would be hurt by the loss of employment, finances, and a social life. His income together with G's was very comfortable, and even without G's contribution he would have an adequate financial status, but he would have to give up his opulent lifestyle. He also saw that although G was determined to have a particular kind of life, it was a better life than the kind F had previously known during his battles with depression.

One of the most interesting aspects of treating F was his desire to talk about the psychological reasons for his behaviors and depression. He had a deep conviction that all his behavior would change and his depression would vanish if he understood his inner conflicts. He remonstrated the therapist regularly for trying to get him to change his behavior without first discussing what the possible psychological causes for the behaviors were. He hated the idea of medication for his depression and felt it was a superficial treatment. He had a deep conviction that all behaviors and feelings that were abnormal were rooted in internal psychological conflicts. On at least one occasion, he said that he understood why one would try a medication or behavioral approach with poor patients who could not afford the kind of treatment that explored their psyche, but he thought it would be better to get at the underlying cause when a patient had the means to do so. He was not chagrined when we pointed out how much he had paid for two years of that kind of explorative therapy with no improvement in his condition, and for at least a year he occasionally tried to direct his treatment along psychological lines only.

In general, in behavioral disorders, why patients do what they do at the beginning of the disorder has little or nothing to do with why they continue the behavior when it becomes an addiction. The factors that *sustain* behavior are different from those that *initiate* it. The desire to find a meaningful understanding of the roots of feelings and actions in this case can be a trap, as they encourage patients with addictive behaviors to search endlessly for the cause without ever having to give up the behaviors that afflict them. A problem of addiction treatment is that the patients hate the consequences but desire the behaviors, and while they discuss the meaning of their behavior, they can continue to engage in it.

In this case, we assured F that we would gladly discuss why he did these things after he stopped. In fact he initially was very interested in this discussion, but later he seemed much less interested in why and more interested in how to stop. Most of our work after he had accepted the diagnosis of paraphilia was directed at how to stop thinking about certain sexual activities, how to avoid triggers that made him crave those behaviors, and how to keep his partner from leaving him.

F was referred for ongoing psychotherapy but was warned that discussion of his cravings and the details of his impulses could ultimately be a trigger for his behavior. The more he focused on what he wanted and had been forced to give up, the more he would resent his partner and the worse his quality of his life would seem. Instead, F was encouraged to focus on the things he had, wanted to keep, and therefore wanted to appreciate. With this in mind, he was a more active participant in his therapy and eventually continued in couples therapy with his partner.

Chapter Seven
Life Story Problems in
the HIV Clinic

Emil Kraepelin's view of psychiatric disorders as diseases was a dominant theme through most of the mid- to late nineteenth century. In the early twentieth century, much of the field of psychiatry turned its attention away from diseases of the brain and toward the internal workings of the mind and the experiences that shape a person's inner life. Psychiatrists began to broaden their views at the behest of many great thinkers, with the work of Adolf Meyer having as much of an effect as that of Sigmund Freud. Meyer believed that one could not understand psychiatry outside the context of a person's narrative life story, and he taught his students to record the lives of their patients during their evaluations. The term *biopsychosocial* has its origins in the work of Meyer and his students.

Meyer contended that to view psychiatric patients purely as the diseases they have would ultimately result in the development of programs to exterminate them. He lived to see the prophetic nature of his ideas as he saw the rise of the eugenics movement in the United States, with the sterilization of mentally infirm persons, and the Nazi extension of eugenics resulting in the efforts to exterminate the mentally ill in Germany. Similar concerns may unfold as we watch the development of assisted suicide programs, the Netherlands' legalization of euthanasia, and the rapid proliferation of programs that essentially ration medical care and carve mental disorders out of payment programs for medical care.

The *Diagnostic and Statistical Manual of Mental Disorders, Fourth Edition* (DSM-IV), a document that is essentially similar to the work of Kraepelin, describes psychiatric disorders as syndromes and diseases. It largely misses the relationship between life experience and the disorder it can cause. In a sense, a disease is a problem of brain, a broken part in the hardware that runs the mind, which is the operating system software. Distortions in programming the mind through adverse experiences confound the operating system. In a sense, the brain is fine, whereas the mind is troubled. This is something of a simplification, as the experiences of life are stored in brain as neuronal change, but substantial experience suggests that the operating system is plastic; that is, it can be repaired by all the forms of psychotherapy that Jerome Frank studied and reported in his groundbreaking book, *Persuasion and Healing.*[1] This chapter describes the interventions that are useful for treating the problems that occur in the lives of persons with HIV.

Individual, Cultural, and Social Assumptions and Disorders Emerging from the Assumptive World

We assume that the way we interpret the world is accurate, and experience dictates much of the way we interpret the world. A clear example is D, the patient from Case 4 who developed pneumonia after a successful detoxification and substantial improvement. We offered to get him a home nebulizer machine to help his condition, but we also asked him what he would be willing to do in exchange for our efforts to get it (we wanted him to volunteer to give up cigarettes). He offered us $50 if we would write the prescription that would allow him to get the machine. When we told him we meant that he give up smoking, he laughed and began to discuss his assumptions about our request that he do something for it. He described bribing police officers, "buying" prescriptions from doctors, and getting paid for a sexual encounter with a counselor in juvenile detention as a teenager. We discussed how his assumptions affected the way he saw his life and life itself.

We live in a world of assumptions. Some emerge from the types of people we are, but many emerge from the experiences we have had and the life we encounter. In patient care, one often has to confront the role that assumptions play in patients' problems and their patterns of behavior. A wonderful line from one of our bright patients is "I inject heroin only two or three times a week; that doesn't make me a junkie." She was living with a boyfriend who was a junkie (using her definition) who hit her regularly and was working two jobs to support his habit. She assumed this was how people lived, as her mother had supported her alcoholic father, and many of her friends and family members lived in similar circumstances.

Assumptions emerge from the individual, the culture, and the society in which we live. Those assumptions change the way we behave. They drive our expectations, our goals, and our view of ourselves. We assume that a behavior such as hard work will result in rewards, or will result in futility; it will allow us to be promoted ahead of others, or it will allow others to take credit for our work and be promoted ahead of us. Within this is buried the simple truth that over time, although our original assumptions are shaped by our experience, our assumptions eventually come to shape our experience. This is a critical point to understand in the world of HIV and psychiatry. Changes in behavior will change the way we encounter the world and finally reshape assumptions. To be able to change assumptions, one must essentially rewrite the operating system of the mind, which will lead to a change in behavior and experience (see Fig. 7.1).

The first step is to identify assumptions. This is why Meyer puts so much emphasis on knowing the patient's life and therefore understanding his or her personal assumptions. Patients who experience childhood sexual misuse at the hands of a parental figure receive a clear message that *feelings direct behavior*. No matter how illicit the behavior is considered, if the feelings are strong enough, it is okay to engage in the behavior. Similar messages come from physical abuse, abusive language, criminal behavior, drug and alcohol abuse, excessive gambling, and other self-indulgent behaviors that can damage the integrity of the family. If this assumption is manifest in a patient, such as the one with strong feelings (D), he or she is more likely to act on those feelings. The more the person acts on feelings, the more chaos he or she encounters in life from further

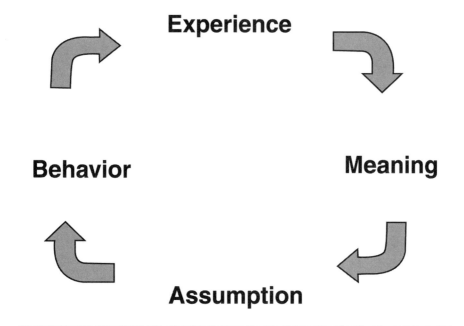

Fig. 7.1. The cycle of life experience

misuse and misadventure. The individual's assumptions become the author of his or her life experience, which further confirms those assumptions.

Cultural and social assumptions have an equivalent effect. The recent emphasis on cultural sensitivity is an example of the power of cultural assumptions in patient care. A patient from the East Baltimore African American community may distrust the medical practices at Johns Hopkins Hospital because of the common beliefs in that community that he or she may be used for medical experiments, misused, and perhaps even killed during their medical care. Patients who come to trust us often share the stories of patients who disappeared into Johns Hopkins never to be heard from again. The tales are apocryphal as our patients admit that they never actually knew the person involved but are certain that the story is true. Such assumptions come to be self-confirming. Patients delay care until desperately ill, coming to the emergency room at the last possible moment, decreasing their likelihood of a good outcome, and making themselves more anonymous to the system.

Our current culture places a premium on self-expression, feelings, self-discovery, and freedom. These are values we share and laud. Not everyone is made worse by these values, and most benefit from them. However, a vulnerable person with major depression is made more vulnerable to suicide by these values. A person with strong feelings and impulses is at a higher risk for letting such feelings run his or her life. An individual with a liability to drug addiction, paraphilia, alcohol abuse, or another disorder of motivated behavior is likely to indulge in that interest. Cultural, social, and individual assumptions may either ameliorate or exacerbate the person's underlying vulnerabilities. For example, the risky behaviors that lead to possible HIV infection can be seen as being encouraged by both individual and cultural assumptions.

Life experiences also cause both positive and negative reinforcement of behavior. In a sense, patients can learn pathological behaviors. Reinforcement may have encouraged these behaviors, and over time the behavior becomes habit. This can lead to a habitual approach to problems that nearly guarantees bad results. The complexity of reinforcement is such that a patient may be conditioned by immediate rewards (such as heroin intoxication) to tolerate much larger punishments (such as poverty, starvation, and homelessness). Eventually, the patient will develop the assumption that this is the way life is supposed to be. This can lead patients to believe that such behaviors are automatic and impossible to change. They say they cannot help it; they feel as if they have no choice and cannot act otherwise.

The synergy between learned life experience and the assumptions made because of experience make change very difficult. One's life course is set in motion and proceeds based on behaviors that emerge from unconscious habits that have been conditioned by rewards and meaningful assumptions that have been shaped by experience. HIV-infected adults who have a history of childhood sexual or physical abuse have reported engaging in more HIV-prone behaviors such as drug abuse and sexual compulsivity than persons with no history of trauma. One useful metaphor follows: "You are on a trail that you have learned to follow, and now you want to set out in a direction where there is no trail." We urge patients to confront their reflexive behavior and to try a new direction, but to also expect slow progress, a return of old habitual responses, and that they might "get lost along the way."

Disruption of Development

Life follows a sequence of development, with cognitive, emotional, and behavioral tasks that must be mastered before a next phase of life can be reached. These tasks have been extensively described in the works of Erik Erikson and many others. The disruption of these sequences creates disorders. The disruption of development affects an individual's assumptions about life, but it also may prevent the development of crucial skills necessary for recovery. A lack of mature coping skills may be a direct consequence of a childhood affective illness that delays development. The social skills needed to recover from an illness, psychological trauma, or adversity may never develop.

Psychotherapy directed at recovery from the disruption of such sequences has been widely discussed, but it usually focuses on the effective modeling of missing skills, education, and cognitive behaviorally directed exercises aimed at mastering particular situations and tasks. However, it is necessary, in order to determine the goals of psychotherapy interventions, to understand how life experiences have caused developmental disruptions. Developmental disruptions will lead to a variety of unlearned skills, so this approach opens the patient up to a more global improvement. This hearkens back to Adolf Meyer and his view that psychiatric disorders can be understood from knowing the patient's personal history.

Demoralization

The kind of depression described in Chapter 2 probably represents the result of a brain disease, but our research suggests that half the patients complaining of "depression" have something that is not a disease. For the sake of discussion, their depression can be called *demoralization*. Demoralization is the psychological state of loss, grief, sadness, and despair that accompanies psychological injuries. It is a universal human experience, found in romantic disappointment, occupational adversity, and most acutely in the death of a parent, spouse, beloved friend, or (for those in medicine) patient. Elizabeth Kübler-Ross described stages of grief in her book, *On Death and Dying*.[2] Although grief is a psychological state that is unpleasant and can diminish functioning, like all life experiences, it is unique to each individual and event.

Most people are impaired by profound grief. Spouses may die after the loss of their partner. Children often miss work at the death of a parent. Some cultures and religions have prescribed periods of grieving during which one expects diminished activity. Often difficulties with sleep, concentration, and memory result. These symptoms should improve over time, but in vulnerable patients symptoms of unresolved demoralization may persist.

Endless examples demonstrate that psychological vulnerabilities make recovery from demoralization chronic and difficult. A patient may discover that he has infected someone he loves at the same time he discovers that he is infected. This can be particularly bad if the person he infected has no risk factors and develops AIDS as the presenting problem. Patients may have to reconsider the lack of control they have had during their lives when they are diagnosed with HIV. Some patients develop AIDS and have difficulty accepting the necessary self-discipline to take antiviral medication. Dealing with disfigurement and body habitus changes can overwhelm patients, particularly those who find their own appearance an important element of their life. Also, unresolved conflicts with people who die may lead to prolonged grief on the part of patients. Those with chronic illness who lose caregivers may experience profound demoralization.

The treatment for demoralization requires therapeutic optimism, support, and time. New coping skills must be learned and old ones improved to effect rehabilitation. The development of these coping skills is based on personality and style, as described in Chapter 4. Patients who are focused on the present may adapt to change quite easily, but they have difficulty with perseverance and discomfort. Future-focused patients may have resilience when it comes to self-discipline, but they may see only the losses of the future looming while being unable to enjoy the pleasures of the present. Whole books have been written on techniques to improve coping skills, and specific literature is available on teaching coping skills to HIV-infected patients. We have found it useful to help patients not only develop their own coping skills but also be able to recognize the situations when they will need coaching from a therapist because of their own vulnerabilities.

The different areas of the demoralized patient's life must be assessed for function and structure. One example would be a detailed inquiry into a patient's employment situation with attention paid to the nature and quality of relationships with coworkers and bosses, the structure of the work environment and schedule, and the patient's assessment of his or her feelings about the work produced. A difference exists between structure and function, but both tend to build on each other. Thus, frequently participating in certain activities helps improve a particular function through practice, while mastery of the function in a specific area of life is likely to improve its frequency. These things must occasionally be prescribed as part of rehabilitation for a demoralized patient. In our occupational example, we might discuss new approaches to handling conflict with a coworker, helping to open the patient to a discussion of the assumptions that color the current problematic approach. Enhancements in a patient's social, occupational, romantic, family, cultural, and recreational life can lead to profound improvements in his or her quality of life and mood.

Psychotherapy for demoralization must be optimistic and founded in experience. Hopeless patients see their problems as intractable; they see no way to improve. A clear discussion of how things are likely to get better, what improvements they can expect over a certain period of time, and what can be done for them to help with those improvements is often overlooked and critical. In working with addicted patients, few can imagine a life without drugs. A description of such a life may remoralize them and increase their motivation for treatment.

The coping strategies for psychiatric conditions such as major depression, schizophrenia, personality disorder, addiction, and chronic medical illness share many similar features. The principles include education, a description of treatment goals, the likely outcome, and an outline for how the psychotherapy will be performed and its rules. Patient role induction is often the most important part of the treatment. Interventions include supportive, cognitive-behavioral, and insight-oriented work, depending on the need of the patient and his or her condition. Patients with psychiatric disorders also become demoralized and need the same kind of treatments described here.

The Trap of Meaning

The currency of the integration of experience, emotion, sensation, and interaction with the world is meaning. What does an experience, a conversation, a feeling, or an injury mean? We wonder what we mean when we say something, do something, or feel something, and we wonder what others mean by their behavior toward us. We make assumptions about what to expect based on what we think an encounter means. Much of the currency of psychiatry lies in the realm of meaning as well. Our assumptions about what things mean are critical to our functioning. We want to know why we are sad, hurt, sick, in pain, or unable to get what we want. The search for meaning helps us survive and predict the future. We wish to know what to expect, and we abstract meaning from our experience to master our environment and improve our circumstances.

The psychological meaning of things has great significance to us. In the twentieth century, a focus on the psychological meanings of behavior and emotion led to assumptions about experience that can be of great use in the treatment of patients. Friedrich Nietzsche was a pioneer in the arena of meaning, but his largest contribution was the cynical idea that occult motivations are self-serving in a way that is greedy, selfish, and base. When you help another, you are inflating your own importance. Charity is an effort to make yourself feel fortunate. Many social critics attributed base occult motivation to behaviors that seemed laudable and altruistic. One of the loudest of these voices was Sigmund Freud, who pioneered the exploration of unconscious drives and wishes as motivators for all psychological problems. Freud believed that unacceptable wishes and desires, particularly those in the domain of sexual and libidinal gratification, were kept unconscious, but they caused conflict that led to psychological symptoms.

The method used by Freud and his disciples attempts to change behaviors by understanding their significance or meaning. If we know why we do a thing, perhaps we can change what we do. Essentially, the goal of this work is to change the feelings attached to behaviors and objects, and so change the behavior in response to them. By understanding your feelings toward them, your feelings may change, and your behavior may also change. This powerful method was found to be useful by many thousands of patients and clinicians over the course of the twentieth century. Although critics have derided the efforts of psychodynamic and psychoanalytic treatment, simply the numbers of patients who felt resoundingly helped and even transformed by this form of treatment should give the critics pause.

The liability of this method is that it can be used to explain anything. We can say that all problems of mental life have origins in adverse experience during development. We can postulate that people have schizophrenia, become alcoholics, or suffer from personality difficulties because of inadequate (or excessive) breast-feeding. Many psychiatric textbooks factually state that panic disorder is caused by coitus interruptus and that panic attacks are a frustrated form of orgasm. Some readers may think we are joking here, but many psychiatrists, psychologists, and other mental health professionals memorized these facts much as one might learn physiology. The classic description of the schizophrenogenic mother, by Fromm-Reichman,[3] might seem funny today, filled as it is with almost baseless certainty, if it were not for the sad fact that psychiatrists told the mothers of schizophrenia patients that they had caused the condition with their parenting style.

Clinicians often try to help patients with an intervention called an interpretation. The essence of an interpretation is "I believe you do this behavior because of this underlying cause or meaning." The goal of the interpretation is to help change the behavior. A simple example is a patient who came for treatment because he had troubles with male authority figures such as bosses and teachers, and he was constantly losing good jobs because of it. In his evaluation he described his father as a terrible bully. At some point in his treatment, after careful evaluation for other conditions, his therapist (GT) suggested that perhaps he experienced male authority figures in the way a helpless child experiences a bullying father. He suggested that the patient might do better if he realized he was a grown peer and was not helpless in the situation. The patient reacted with considerable irritation and said, "You're saying I act like a child?"

The therapist quickly said that that was not exactly what he meant (noticing that he himself might be considered a male authority figure by the patient) and tried to explain his meaning, causing further irritation. In a much later session, the patient said that he realized that all his friends at work also had problems with his boss, so he had started to copy the behavior of the employees who got along with his boss, and that this was solving his problem. In an even later session he referred back to the original interpretation and said, "I wasn't acting like a helpless child; I was acting like my father."

Three interpretations arose during the sessions with this patient, and one might ask which one is correct. It is more useful, however, when using the life-story method to ask which interpretation was the most effective in helping to change the patient's behavior. Jerome Frank might say that the goal of any therapy is not to make the right interpretation, but the one that helps the patient heal and be persuaded to change. The hazard of interpretation is the relentless search for meaning without any action on the patient's part to change as the understanding of the underlying meaningful connections grows. The impressive power of the life-story method application flows from the well-constructed interpretations that provoke change.

A second example is a patient seen for evaluation because of copraphagia (eating feces). This pleasant woman came complaining of medical problems but quickly admitted that if she had a bowel movement before she was ready, she ate it to punish herself for not being able to hold it. She had been in treatment for the problem for many years, and when asked what she discussed in her sessions, she said she discussed why she did it. She was encouraged to stop discussing why she did it and instead discuss how to stop doing it. In her case, she had become trapped in the search for the meaning of her behavior and assumed that as soon as she understood why she did it, she would stop doing it.

The other trap of meaning is that meaningful hypotheses cannot be proved or disproved and therefore may prevent patients from receiving treatment for other disorders. An example is a patient who was admitted to the ward at Johns Hopkins with HIV, depression, and suicidal feelings. He had been persuaded by another therapist that his depression was the result of ego dystonic (internal conflict about and nonacceptance of) homosexuality, and that he would get better if he could just accept himself as he was or limit himself to heterosexual activity.

When we pointed out to him that he had not been depressed until about a year before he was admitted despite his lifelong sexual preference, he replied that he had been in denial of his feelings before he became depressed. Ultimately, he accepted treatment with antidepressants, but as his depression resolved he explained that he thought he had improved because we had "gratified his desire for the sick role," and that by swallowing his medication he was symbolically "swallowing his doctor."

The resident on the case asked how we knew that we were pursuing the correct treatment. One explanation we provided was that nortriptyline worked for depression in controlled trials against placebo treatment because it tastes exactly like a doctor, and that placebo tastes like something else. The resident laughed at this but saw the issue that the patient's hypotheses were not testable and resulted in a treatment impasse. It is possible, by the way, that the patient was correct, and the success of the medication in this patient was based on its meaning instead of its action in the brain, and this may, in fact, explain the placebo response phenomenon seen in some patients in clinical trials.

Meanwhile, in the process of awaiting evidence for this hypothesis, we continue to recommend that clinicians try to distinguish between the disorders that originate in the meanings that patients create about the world based on their experience and the diseases of brain that confound their perceptions of the world.

Post-Traumatic Stress Disorder (PTSD)

Traumatic events that are life threatening provoke terror, anxiety, and stress in most people. In some individuals, the chronicity, intensity, frequency, and comorbidity of these symptoms can become psychiatrically disabling. Specifically, patients may have intrusive intense recollections of the traumatic event, sometimes to the point where they feel as if they are experiencing the event again. Patients will persistently avoid stimuli associated with the trauma and display persistent symptoms of increased arousal not present before the trauma, such as hypervigilance, an exaggerated startle response, and feelings of anticipation of a negative experience. When these symptoms persist for more than one month and interfere with social, familial, and/or occupational functioning, the term *post-traumatic stress disorder* (PTSD) is used to designate the disordering nature of the reaction. PTSD has a current prevalence of less than 1 percent and a lifetime prevalence of 1–9 percent with a female-to-male lifetime prevalence ratio of 2:1. Rape is the traumatic event most likely to produce PTSD outside of military settings, particularly if it occurs before or during adolescence.[4] PTSD is associated with an increased likelihood of engaging in destructive behaviors such as alcohol and other drug abuse, sexual promiscuity, or prostitution.

Symptoms of PTSD have been associated with HIV risk behaviors and HIV progression. Prostitution, injection drug use, and choosing high-risk sex partners have all been behaviors common to young adults whose PTSD symptoms began during adolescence. In one study, 42 percent of HIV-infected women presented evidence of PTSD,[5] and veterans with PTSD are at increased risk for HIV infection. Women prisoners with a lifetime history of PTSD are more likely to have engaged in prostitution and receptive anal intercourse before incarceration compared to women prisoners without PTSD.[6] It is possible that PTSD increases the risk for HIV, but it is also possible that HIV risk behaviors, such as prostitution or drug abuse, increase exposure to trauma and thus the likelihood of developing PTSD. Alternatively, PTSD that stems from early trauma may predispose an individual to engage in sex or drug behaviors that can increase the risk of HIV infection.

The presence of PTSD in an at-risk or HIV-positive individual is of particular concern because of high rates of comorbidity (up to 80 percent) with other psychiatric disorders. Specifically, PTSD is most often comorbid with depression and cocaine/opioid abuse,[7] both risk factors for HIV. Prior depression may be either a risk factor for the development of PTSD following a traumatic event or a co-occurring response with PTSD to a trauma. Substance abuse may be either an attempt to self-medicate the experience of suffering after a traumatic experience or a lifestyle that increases exposure to traumatic events, such as robbery or assault.[8]

PTSD and substance use disorders that occur together can adversely affect treatment. Comorbid conditions have been associated with poorer treatment adherence and motivation, quicker relapse, more inpatient hospitalizations and medical problems, and lower global functioning than either disorder alone.[9] Thus, treatment of PTSD that does not address coexisting depression or substance abuse may be insufficient or even worsen a patient's psychiatric status. Any individuals presenting with symptoms of PTSD should routinely be screened for depression and substance use disorders. For HIV-infected individuals with PTSD and another concurrent psychiatric disorder, treatment that simultaneously addresses both disorders is likely to be more effective and practical.

The treatment of PTSD is quite controversial in the current literature. PTSD is a condition that may remain problematic for patients for long periods of time. We emphasize a careful evaluation for other psychiatric conditions, role induction into treatment, and the avoidance of benzodiazepine use. Pharmacological treatment with antidepressants has been helpful in our experience and has extensive evidence for efficacy, particularly the SSRI antidepressants. In our experience, patients seem to respond best to treatments that emphasize rehabilitation and function, as opposed to those that focus on the meaningful issues of the trauma. Addressing substance use, personality disorder, and major depression in patients with PTSD is essential to an effective treatment.

Special Therapy Issues for the HIV Clinic

Life with HIV is filled with difficult, special problems for patients. Good clinicians must know the essential principles of delivering bad news and of counseling patients who are at risk, who test positive, and who test negative. Fear of HIV infection may lead patients with no real risk to come for repeated testing. Such patients may have obsessive-compulsive disorder and other anxiety conditions. It is important to recognize such patients and help them receive appropriate treatment.

The principles of discussing any medical problem are all applicable to HIV testing and counseling. Each patient needs to understand the potential risks and benefits of the procedure, the role of the clinician, and his or her own responsibilities in the process. The clinician should describe what will happen in the event of a positive test and then be prepared to help the patient if the test is positive. Make extra time available for a positive result in order to educate the patient and present him or her with a plan for treatment.

Pretest, Test, and Post-test Counseling and Education

Patients at risk for HIV infection are often reticent to be tested. Surveys suggest they fear the results of the test or are too overwhelmed by the issues of their current lives and behaviors to present for testing. Before 1993, patients who received a positive HIV test result saw their diagnosis as essentially fatal. Additionally, many patients thought it would be burdensome to know that they were placing others at risk for infection. In more recent years with the advent of highly active antiretroviral therapy (HAART), HIV has become a chronic treatable illness. In this setting, it seems more reasonable for patients to be tested and engage in treatment. Nonetheless, survey data show that a large number of patients who are at significant risk are not being tested. Psychoeducational psychotherapy directed at encouraging patients to be tested has been offered to a variety of at-risk populations. The outcomes of these intervention studies show that such psychotherapy does result in patients being tested and diagnosed earlier.

The current protocol for testing HIV-infected patients involves an initial enzyme-linked immunoabsorbent assay (ELISA) that detects antibodies made by the patient in response to the HIV virus. Because this test has false positives, before notifying a patient of a positive test result, a confirmation is made using a second technique to detect HIV antibodies called a Western blot. Both of these tests look for antibodies and therefore, immediately after infection when patients have not yet developed antibodies to HIV, these tests will be negative despite the fact that the patient is infected.

Pretest counseling has been described in a number of papers. Before testing, patients must give informed consent to have the test performed. Much has been written on the medico-legal concept of informed consent in many other works, but in essence it involves providing the patient with information regarding the meaning of positive and negative tests, so that he or she can make an informed decision about having the test and interpreting the results. It should be stressed that a negative test does not mean that a patient is immune and cannot become infected later, and that a positive result does not mean that a person has AIDS, is going to die, or will have opportunistic infections. It should also be emphasized that the test will remain negative for a time after infection (the time it takes for antibodies to develop), and therefore after a recent exposure, a patient may have a negative test but in fact be infected. Pretest counseling should also cover safer sex, safe needle use, and other risk-reduction interventions, because a significant percentage of patients who obtain testing return much later for their results and sometimes not at all.

Post-test counseling issues include psychoeducational interventions regarding the meaning of test results, recommendations for treatment, and, importantly, risk-reduction interventions to stem the spread of HIV infection. These post-test interventions should occur in both HIV-negative and HIV-positive patients.

At the time patients are given their test results, it is not uncommon for them to have a variety of intense psychological reactions, including suicidal feelings, anger, homicidal thoughts directed at potentially infecting partners, overwhelming grief, and a complete psychological breakdown. Patients with poor coping skills, poor impulse control, a history of suicidal feelings and behaviors, substance abuse disorders, and a lack of social supports are at an increased risk for impulsive or self-destructive behaviors. Because of these circumstances, the availability of psychological interventions at the time of HIV testing and result provision is critical.

Although a separate matter, bad news regarding the progression of the HIV infection can provoke similar responses in patients and probably should be considered in a similar way. The transition from the asymptomatic phase to the development of an opportunistic infection or to a formal diagnosis of AIDS because of a decline in CD4 cells may provoke the same reactions as those described previously. Again, the presence of psychological and intervention is extremely critical in this setting. Patients may be overwhelmed by the news that they need to start antiretroviral drugs and therefore need emergent attention at this time.

Perhaps the most difficult event for a newly diagnosed patient is the disclosure of the illness to friends, family, and partners. Social stigma and fears of abandonment may play a role in making this difficult, and an embarrassment over the risk behaviors and route of transmission also clearly plays a role. Complicating this is the issue of infectious transmission to partners, who may or may not be aware of the risky behavior that caused the infection in the first place. HIV clinicians often play an important role in helping and coaching patients regarding the disclosure of this information. It is essential that patients be counseled about the need to notify and test those at risk. It is also important to help them deal with the very real stigma of the diagnosis of HIV. Despite public education about the lack of casual transmission of HIV, significant fear and anxiety still exists in the general public about contact with infected persons. It is common for patients to have difficulty at work, at home, and in social situations. Some are told they cannot have contact with children in their families, and some are asked not to have contact with their families at all. It can be a difficult time for patients, and support is often crucial.

The landmark legal decision in the 1976 Tarasoff case in California has redefined the role and responsibility of clinicians in relationship to confidentiality. In the case, a psychiatrist was found to have had a duty to warn a third-party victim, because he knew his patient intended to harm that party. Until that time, physicians felt bound by confidentiality, but it is a reasonable argument that preventing a patient from committing a murder is in the patient's best interest. A variety of legislation differing from state to state has afforded practitioners an increased number of options with regard to confidential situations. In some states, Tarasoff statutes (which establish the duty to warn vulnerable individuals of imminent danger from a patient, overriding issues of confidentiality) have completely changed the way in which mental health professionals handle confidential issues.

It is a similar argument that it is equally in a patient's interest to prevent him or her from transmitting HIV to a potential contact. Numerous articles have been written about the issues of ethics, confidentiality, the duty to warn, and the medical/legal aspects of this element of practice. Although no clear consensus has been reached, it has been recommended that patients who are sexually active and infected with HIV be counseled about potential risks to their sexual partners. Additionally, known partners should be notified of exposure risks and potential infections as well. Partner notification has been an extremely hotly debated topic; however, many states have developed legislation requiring or allowing either physicians or health department officials to notify partners of HIV-infected patients of their risk. The current standard, despite the controversy, appears to be an obligation on the part of health care professionals to notify anyone clearly identifiable who could be construed to be at risk and yet unaware of it.

A particularly difficult situation is that of sex workers known to be HIV-infected and working actively as prostitutes. Public opinion of prostitution shapes the way in which this particular problem is addressed in any given area and may significantly reduce the availability of testing and treatment for sex workers and their sex partners, who may be described alternatively as clients, customers, victims, or victimizers, depending on who is doing the describing. The response to this problem has ranged from the view that sex care workers and their clients can make their own decisions and should be responsible for their own behavior, all the way to the sentiment that sex workers and/or partners should be arrested and jailed for attempted murder. Also, sex workers are impaired by a variety of psychiatric conditions, including cognitive impairment, major mental illness, personality disorder, and substance use disorders. These may further contribute to the sense that some sex workers may be less than fully responsible for their behavior. Recommendations have been made for voluntary and involuntary interventions regarding these patients. A psychiatric intervention for these individuals may involve assessing their capacity to make medical decisions or understand the informed consent process. Treatments for the conditions that impair these patients are also critical to reining in the spread of the epidemic.

Facing Death and Severe Illness

Since the revolution in treatment for HIV that began when HAART became the standard of care, the number of HIV-related deaths has diminished remarkably. Consequently, the special AIDS hospices and nursing homes that proliferated in the early 1990s have become uncommon. This improvement in outcome provides little comfort to those patients who are dying of AIDS, and still a great need exists for expertise in helping patients and their families cope with grief and end-of-life issues. One of the identified problems of this phase of care is the sense of abandonment that many patients describe as those close to them see them becoming ill and infirm. Unfortunately, health care providers who become "burned out" and quit are no longer able to serve this community of patients who desperately need them, as the valuable expertise the providers have developed is then lost to those dealing with feelings of abandonment. This means that each provider must know his or her limitations and hone their skills when working with very ill patients.

As patients become ill, they often need significant support from their physicians and care providers, and this may influence providers to promise more than they can truly deliver. It is better to give in a limited way that is consistent and sustained than to promise everything and later need to abandon the patient to survive. Even patients in the terminal stages of an illness appear to benefit from a care plan detailing the specific palliative therapies that will be used. Therapeutic optimism and hope are also a continued part of the care of terminally ill patients.

Therapy for dying patients still involves assessments for other conditions, such as depression and delirium, but it mostly consists of adequate medication for comfort and symptom relief, as well as talk therapy focused on the issues raised by the patient. A discussion of what the patient prefers during the terminal phase of care is necessary, but the dialog should be continued as the condition progresses and appropriate education is reinforced. Many patients have strong preconceived notions of what they want and do not want done for them, but these are often based on limited experience and knowledge. It is common for patients to tell us they never want to be placed on mechanical ventilation, only to change their minds when they develop air hunger. Many patients have later told us that they were grateful for the opportunity to change their minds.

Significant pressure is being placed on the current health care system to do less for patients in an effort to decrease the cost and expenditure of resources. The pressure from health care administration is predominantly felt by physicians and their colleagues. Patients also feel this pressure and may make decisions to terminate care at a particular point that is premature and even inappropriate because of this pressure. Vulnerable people are more easily manipulated in this way; therefore, those most knowledgeable about their condition should function as their advocates.

When patients describe what they want for care at the end of life, they talk about communication, accessibility, symptom relief, support, and practitioner expertise. Some authors have criticized research around medical choices at the end of life, pointing out that much of the research is biased by the attitudes of the researchers.[10] We have often seen patients who would gladly trade choice and autonomy for comfort and guidance. Patients seldom understand the choices they are asked to make and want clear recommendations as well as help with making the decisions.

Support and education are important interventions for patients with a serious illness. Group treatment, including group education and support, can often be a useful means for providing this care, and it may help patients cope with problems more effectively than if they only received individual attention. Peer education and support can often be more directive and supportive than that coming from a clinician. Many of our patients have found that the subjective experience of their illness is improved through their involvement in group support. Additionally, confrontation by group members may lead to improved health-directed behaviors and may even change the course for some patients who have not pursued antiviral treatment.

Facing Life after Facing Death

An issue common to the field between 1996 and 1998 was that of facing life after facing death. We had many patients who had exhausted resources in the expectation of death (a process referred to by insurers as "spending down"), become disabled, made plans for their own death, and dealt with issues of loss and dying, only to find themselves remarkably well after the initiation of HAART. Several papers described this phenomenon, in which bewildered and demoralized patients faced the seemingly overwhelming task of rehabilitation and restarting their lives.[11] We have seen a number of these patients, and some still come for care as they recover from long illnesses and gradually regain their strength and initiative. Although this is a problem for fewer people, the effects of new treatments hold not only hope and promise for the future but also challenges for the patient. Clinicians must be able to catalyze such changes and help patients face their new challenges.

Chapter Eight
Special Problems:
Hepatitis C and Adherence

Psychiatric Vectors of Infectious Disease and Hepatitis C Infection

The fundamental thesis of this book is that disorders driven by behavior are more frequent in vulnerable patients than other groups. This phenomenon is exaggerated when the factors driving infection are identified and those at risk are warned to modify their behavior. The current epidemics of HIV, hepatitis C, syphilis, gonorrhea, and even tuberculosis are variously affected by these circumstances. Tuberculosis has the fewest behavioral elements involved directly in the process of infection, but psychiatric disorders lead to an increased risk of exposure and a decreased likelihood of detection and treatment. Rates of tuberculosis infection are higher for those with chronic mental illness, addiction, institutionalization, poverty, substance abuse, and homelessness.

Although this book is devoted to the relationship between HIV and psychiatric disorders, hepatitis C has become an increasing focus of our work. The fundamental principles described in this book could alternately apply to hepatitis C, as it has many of the same characteristics as HIV with regards to risky behaviors. The data for the relationship between hepatitis C and psychiatric disorders have not been extensively researched, but many parallels exist in terms of both behavioral risks for infection and decreased access to treatment. Although, as of this writing, the largest group of HIV-infected patients remains those whose risk category is men who have sex with men, the group with the highest rate of new cases of HIV has become injecting drug users (IDUs). Hepatitis C has undergone a similar epidemic change. Twenty years ago, patients were unknowingly infected mostly through transfusions and less by other means. Now the primary route of infection is injection drug use by a large margin. Our

HIV clinic has a very high rate of coinfection. It was estimated that 4 million people are infected with hepatitis C in the United States,[1] about four times as many as are infected with HIV.

Many persons with hepatitis C are unaware of their infection for many years until it is discovered incidentally. Those coinfected with HIV, however, are more likely to progress to liver failure and death. Fig. 8.1 shows the epidemiological pattern of hepatitis C progression in patients without HIV infection. As can be seen in the figure, unlike those with HIV, many patients with hepatitis C never develop clinical disease and can be chronically infected carriers without ever requiring treatment. This makes the issues of treatment complicated, and these issues will be briefly discussed.

Hepatitis C is a condition found at alarming rates in people vulnerable to risk behaviors similar to those of HIV: patients with chronic mental illness,[2] major depression,[3,4] intravenous drug use, alcoholism, and most likely personality disorder. All these conditions can be daunting to the average primary care provider, who is likely to have patients with these conditions even if he or she is not an expert in their treatment, but they are even more daunting to the subspecialist

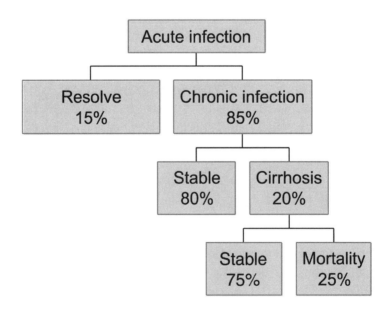

Fig. 8.1. The natural history of hepatitis C infection

Source: Data from Seef LB 1999. Natural history of hepatitis C. *Am J Med* 27, 107(6B):10S–15S.

who is not in the habit of delivering primary care. This leads to a decrease in the likelihood that those with mental illness and hepatitis C will be evaluated and is a barrier to ongoing treatment.

The treatment of hepatitis C is complicated. Currently, the best option for treatment is the use of a combination of ribavirin and interferon, usually given as a fixed-dose combination drug and involving a polyethylene glycol-linked interferon (PEG-interferon or pegylated-interferon). This combination dramatically reduces the amount of hepatitis C virus in the blood and ongoing injury to liver tissue. Ideally, the drugs are given for 24 to 48 weeks, depending on the subtype of hepatitis C virus, and during this time viral replication is inhibited. Unlike HIV, if replication is inhibited completely, some patients will completely clear hepatitis C from their body and have a cure. Several factors influence the cure rate, including the viral subtype, the duration of infection, and the ability to tolerate treatment. Even in the absence of a cure, damage to the liver is reduced during treatment. Different viral subtypes have different rates of response to the drug, but the viral type most prevalent in the United States, type 1, can be cured by treatment about 40 percent of the time in a patient without HIV infection or other serious complications.

Some debate surrounds which patients should receive treatment. Because disease progression does not occur in all patients, some clinicians wait to begin treatment until evidence of liver damage appears on a biopsy. Others strongly favor treating all patients because of high cure rates in early infections. Arguments for delaying treatment include, among others, the long duration, inconvenience, and significant discomfort and side effects of the treatment, including severe psychiatric disturbances. Arguments for an early treatment include the finding that hepatitis C does not seem to develop resistance to interferon, and a treatment trial for several months can predict the likelihood of a cure. In addition, an early treatment provides a hope that all patients can be cured and a decreased likelihood of spreading the infection.

The psychiatric morbidity of treatment with interferon is significant. Mood changes including depression, irritability, anxiety, and fatigue are common during treatment. Patients also complain of decreased concentration, disrupted sleep, and an inability to function. Estimates on the rates of interferon-induced major depression suggest that a third or more patients may develop depression from treatment[5] and that patients are at an increased risk for suicide. Some authors have gone as far as to advocate for prophylactic antidepressant treatment, and a double-blind trial of paroxetine reported a successful reduction in the amount of depression caused by interferon treatment.[6]

The effect of both the prevalence of preexisting psychiatric disorders and the increased risk of developing them when treated with interferon has made it difficult for patients to get treatment if they have comorbid psychiatric disorders. Unfortunately, patients coinfected with HIV and hepatitis C are more likely to develop liver disease, cirrhosis, and liver failure. Although infectious disease subspecialists who treat HIV have had two decades to develop skills in primary care and psychiatric care, gastroenterologists and hepatologists (who provide the majority of hepatitis C care) now need to acquire the skills needed to treat chronically ill patients with comorbid substance use, personality disorder, and major depression. The need for psychiatric expertise has presented a significant barrier to treatment. Unfortunately, this is currently unavailable for the most troubled populations infected with hepatitis C.

Data suggest that other infectious epidemics may have psychiatric vectors as well. Certainly, other sexually transmitted diseases (STDs) fall into this category. We believe that tuberculosis and other infections associated with poverty, exposure, institutionalization, and social and psychological dysfunctions should be considered. At a time when the highest standard of living in the history of humankind is enjoyed in the United States, the radical restructuring of psychiatric treatment to stop this vector of epidemics needs to become a priority.

Adherence to HIV Medications

Although a discussion of adherence is pertinent to many conditions in medicine, it is an issue of great importance to infectious diseases, because imperfect adherence to treatments is one mechanism whereby resistant strains of infectious agents develop. HIV is currently treated with antiretroviral agents that block the actions of specific enzymes that are necessary for the interpretation of HIV ribonucleic acid (RNA) and the production of infectious virions. Genetic mutations of HIV occur spontaneously and frequently. A great many mutations are silent; that is, they produce an HIV particle that is less able to function or ceases the production of an essential product, such that the virion produced is no longer viable. The troublesome mutations are those that alter the reverse transcriptase or protease enzymes slightly but significantly, so that the antiviral drugs cannot bind to them and inhibit their action. This mutant virus is able to continue propagation in the presence of antiviral medications. A wild-type virus, or the virus as it evolves in the absence of antiviral drugs, has the best ability to infect and reproduce in the host. A mutant virus is usually less well adapted and will not survive unless an antiviral drug is present. This means that ideally patients take either no antiviral drug or take a sufficient antiviral drug to completely stop viral replication and prevent mutations from developing.

Perfect adherence increases the likelihood that the medications will suppress the formation of the virus almost completely and thus allow the body's defenses

an advantage in the fight against HIV. With current treatment, HIV is not erad-
icated from the body, but with ideal adherence, viral production is nearly completely suppressed and the disease process can be interrupted, perhaps
indefinitely.

The first patients treated with antiretroviral medications received a single
agent, zidovudine, because that was the only agent available. It was quickly discovered, however, that spontaneous mutations led to HIV strains that had less
sensitivity to zidovudine[7] in patients treated for six months or more. Such evidence led to the development of combination therapy for HIV now commonly
known as highly active antiretroviral therapy, or HAART. By using multiple
agents, the rate of viral replication is slowed so much that few mutations occur,
and mutations that allow resistance to one agent do not protect the virus from
another agent's effect. To be resistant to three agents, many mutations of exactly
the right type would have to occur simultaneously, an event that would be very
unlikely during low rates of viral replication. At high rates of replication, the
number of mutations increases and resistance to any regimen develops.

Studies have shown that the likelihood of a sustained, undetectable viral load
varies directly with adherence to treatment. Ninety-five percent adherence produces about 80 percent effective sustained suppression. There has been substantial debate about the effect of adherence on treatment failure, but an elegant
study of prisoners showed that directly observed therapy under controlled conditions using an intent-to-treat analysis produced an overall rate of 85 percent
undetectable viral loads with prisoners taking about 93 percent of doses.[8] It is
now widely accepted that one must have at least 90–95 percent adherence to
HAART to achieve ideal sustained viral suppression.[9,10]

With the evidence that HAART works well to suppress HIV, and with the
potential danger of viral resistance looming behind every missed dose, one might
find it inconceivable that anyone would have less than perfect adherence to
HAART. Unfortunately, this is not the case for a great many patients. In a recent
British study of antiviral use by community health care providers, it was noted
that only 42 percent of treatment-naive patients achieved undetectable viral
loads.[11] The authors studied the choice of medications and concluded that this
was not the problem. The problem was that many patients did not take their
medications accurately enough to achieve the maximum benefit. Early studies of
adherence focused on the demographic characteristics of patients, and most
were unable to show any effect on patient outcome. In some studies, there is a
trend toward improved adherence in male sex, white ethnicity, older age, higher
income and education, and literacy.[12,13] The literature on adherence, both from
older studies in other conditions and those looking directly at HIV, reveal many
factors that lead to nonadherence, and they can be described in four main

groups: environmental factors, treatment factors, illness factors, and patient factors. The first three groups of factors have a modest effect on adherence, but the last group, patient factors, has been shown to have a remarkable effect on adherence, particularly the psychiatric disorders discussed in the following section.

Environmental factors that contribute to nonadherence include medication cost, work schedules, transportation, housing issues, and the lack of supportive relationships. Missed appointments are a strong predictor of treatment failure, suggesting that any factor that interferes with patients coming for treatment will interfere with adherence.[14] The clinical setting is important, and patient survey data suggest that the patient-provider relationship affects adherence.[15,16] Some insurance plans require the use of a single contracted pharmacy. If this is not conveniently located, it will have a negative influence on patient adherence. Patients' work schedules may interfere with follow-up appointments as well as getting and taking medication. This is even more important if medications produce side effects that interfere with patients' performance at work. Some patients may not have reliable transportation to appointments or to their pharmacy. Homeless patients may have great difficulty storing medicines and may be at the mercy of a friend or relative for transportation or access to their medications. Some patients are alone in the world, and it has been shown that the lack of supportive relationships has a negative influence on adherence.

Most environmental barriers to adherence can, and usually are, overcome through the efforts of the treatment team. These factors are easily assessed when discussing a patient's readiness to start treatment. Once barriers are identified, plans to prevail over them can be easily constructed.

Treatment factors clearly affect adherence, and the choice of treatment often determines the barriers that must be overcome. In general, once-a-day medicines are easier to remember to take regularly than twice-daily medicines, but both are markedly better for adherence than medications that must be taken three or more times daily[12] (middle-of-the-day doses are often missed). Some studies, however, have not seen any effect of pill burden (the number of pills) on adherence.[13] The perceived side effects of treatment also correlate with poor adherence. Patients who believe their treatment causes side effects are more likely to miss doses. There is also clearly less adherence to inconvenient treatment regimens. If a medication needs to be taken with food, without food, no sooner than two hours after a different medication, and so on, patients may have difficulty fitting the pill into their schedules. The more medicines and pills someone takes, the more likely they are to miss doses. Last, patients are less likely to adhere to regimens if they believe them to be ineffective. A belief that treatment is helping improves adherence. Once again, these barriers to adherence can be assessed before treatment and at every follow-up visit, and plans can be formed to tailor treatment to the patient.

Additionally, several factors about an illness have been shown to negatively affect adherence, particularly chronicity, symptoms, and curability. Lifelong illnesses have the highest degree of nonadherence. Illnesses that are asymptomatic often are associated with poor adherence, because the patient is unable to feel any effect from taking a medication. Similarly, illnesses that cause symptoms that are unrelieved by treatment are often associated with poor adherence, as patients are unable to detect a benefit from the medications. Last, illnesses that have no potential cure may lead to a scenario in which the patient is taking treatments that ultimately will fail.

Substantial research has been conducted on what drives better outcomes in chronic diseases that share the same characteristics as HIV, such as hypertension, diabetes, renal failure, and cancer. A central factor is the therapeutic optimism practiced by health care professionals. Health care providers who are willing to explore patients' feelings regarding these issues, who remain supportive, and who emphasize positive outcomes associated with treatment often have better adherence from patients. Therapeutic nihilism has many vocal supporters, including those who guard the health care dollar, autonomy advocates, and "right-to-die" proponents. They focus their arguments on the ideas that all treatments are expensive, burdensome, and ultimately futile (we all die anyway). Therapeutic nihilism is the ultimate in nonadherence—it is nonadherence before the treatment starts. When faced with a chronic, symptomatic, incurable illness, therapeutic optimism can help patients achieve life goals despite illness and treatment.

The patient factors that have the most negative effect on adherence are discussed throughout this book. Early studies of adherence in HIV patients have shown that depression, psychological distress, and substance use (including alcohol) are all associated with poor adherence. Nowhere is this more evident than in the studies showing decreased adherence to HAART caused by depression.[17] Patients with depression are hopeless, care less for themselves, have difficulty with concentration and memory, and experience pain and suffering more acutely. Patients with depression are delayed in receiving HAART[18] and have decreased survival.[19]

Other psychiatric disorders also affect adherence. Substance users are often delayed in receiving HAART, perhaps in an attempt to improve readiness to adherence by achieving long-term abstinence.[18] Psychotic patients with schizophrenia or bipolar mania may refuse to believe they are ill or accept medications, and patients with dementia may not be able to remember to take their medicines.

All patients have the potential for rehabilitation and adherence. Diseases such as major depression, bipolar disorder, schizophrenia, and other chronic mental illnesses all disrupt functioning and imperil patient adherence. Certain efficacious medications and therapies address a wide range of symptoms resulting from psychiatric disorders, and psychiatric care providers can be essential team members in readying a patient for HAART.

Temperamental vulnerabilities also lead to nonadherence. Patients with a high degree of unstable extraversion are motivated by present feelings and immediate rewards more than by the fear of a negative future outcome. They are unable to tolerate discomfort now to avoid consequences in the future. Translated into adherence terms, these patients may quickly abort a treatment if it causes an uncomfortable side effect, or if symptoms resolve and they no longer perceive a need for medications. Asymptomatic illnesses are especially difficult for unstable extraverts, as they must endure treatments that are uncomfortable for no clear "feeling better" reward. For extreme extraverts, the discomfort may be as slight as swallowing a pill, because any discomfort is difficult for them to tolerate. Further, unstable extraverts tend to have pervasively chaotic lives, with little stability to be found in any arena. Such instability does not lend itself to a triumph over the environmental, treatment, and illness barriers to adherence. In some cases, the patient is so feeling-driven as to miss the point of treatment entirely, asking for symptom alleviation for problems caused by his or her own nonadherence behavior.

Adherence training for patients with these vulnerabilities requires constant and consistent coaching. As stated in Chapter 4, the treatment team should clarify the goals of treatment, both short and long term, exchange interventions for desired behaviors, and anticipate misunderstandings driven by feelings. *Role induction* is the psychotherapeutic term applied to the process of teaching the patient how to be a patient. In patients with unstably extraverted temperamental vulnerabilities, this may require a great many encounters. With time, it is useful to demonstrate the rewards of adherence to treatment, no matter how small, and point out the benefits possible with adherence to additional treatments: "Look how great things are now that your mother has let you live in the house again. And all for simply coming to clinic once a week to meet with the therapist! You know, I bet we could get you feeling even better if you took this medicine every day."

Furthermore, addictions are disordering and impair adherence to other pursuits. Active alcohol and other substance use have been shown to have a negative effect on adherence.[20-22] However, simply trading a disordered addiction to heroin for an orderly addiction to methadone can markedly improve adherence to other treatments, such as psychotherapy. Substance intoxication impairs some adherence, but detoxified patients can be induced through rehabilitative therapies to maintain abstinence, and then the principles of adherence to the abstinence program can be applied to other things, such as taking medication. In some cases, addiction treatments like methadone can be tied to other treatments to increase the adherence to the other behavior. Once again, the reader is referred to Chapter 5 and the argument of finding the motivation that will reinforce the desired behavior.

Last, demoralization leads to nonadherence, as stated in Chapter 7, whereas remoralization, through therapeutic optimism, improves adherence. Insights gained by patients regarding their roles in or maladaptive responses to the disorder they encounter can promote health, productivity, and functioning, all of which promote adherence.

Current HIV literature focuses on many of the factors discussed in this chapter. Many papers address the environmental, illness, and treatment factors that have an effect on adherence, yet not much literature has been published on the most profound barriers to adherence: patients' psychiatric conditions. The development of a therapeutic alliance between the patient and health care provider, with the goal of effective therapies for disorder and illness, is the central factor in successful treatment. A rational approach to diagnosis is the first step in this process, and we have attempted to describe throughout this book the way to initiate treatment with patients. Ultimately, the integration of psychiatric services with the care of HIV-infected patients will be the factor that improves adherence for most patients.

Chapter Nine
How to Fight AIDS

In this book, we have described the role of psychiatric disorders in both the dissemination of HIV and the obstruction of effective treatment. We have also described how HIV infection can exacerbate and even cause psychiatric disorders. This cycle is a part of the driving force of the HIV epidemic and is a crucial factor that must be addressed as we advocate for effective treatment.

We present an integrated treatment approach at the beginning of this chapter, followed by a model for the provision of this approach, and finally we will discuss the need for advocacy in the case of mentally ill persons.

An Integrated Approach to Treatment

The treatment of complicated patients requires a determination of what is wrong, a treatment plan to remedy the problem(s), and a therapeutic alliance between the health care team and the patient. Standard medical education stresses the process of looking for a single pathological explanation for all presenting symptoms. In complicated cases, however, a multilateral approach is required, which standard psychiatric education calls the *formulation*. After the development of a differential diagnosis, the various factors contributing to the patient's problems are combined in a formulation that should adequately explain all the problems with which the patient is struggling.

In this book, we have already laid out a logical framework for the formulation of problem factors by the sequence of the disorders discussed. The first step is to consider the disease states that must be treated, as well as both the symptomatic and therapeutic treatments available for each. These include medical diseases (such as HIV, venereal infections, hepatitis C, and various opportunistic infections) and psychiatric disease states (such as major depression, bipolar disease, and schizophrenia).

The second part of the formulation is to consider the dispositional or dimensional elements of the patient. We often use the word *endowments* for these personal traits. Intelligence, temperament, and even immune competence can be considered part of the dimensional formulation. This aspect of a case colors the type of interventions needed for patients and the degree of resources that must be committed for a successful treatment. Understanding the nature of a person's nonengagement in treatment is critical to success in overcoming barriers to adherence. Patients who are cognitively limited may simply need more education, whereas someone who is emotionally unstable may need therapy directed at his or her vulnerabilities. This is similar to the appreciation of the patients' immune state, their nutritional state, and their functional state when considering medical treatment. Patients with poor nutrition may not be able to tolerate rigorous medical interventions until they have been prepared with parenteral nutrition. Those with a personality disorder may need significant therapeutic coaching before they are ready to accept a therapeutic alliance. Personality features also help the clinician to understand the limitations of treatment for a particular patient and why the alliance is uneasy.

The third step in the formulation is the consideration of patient behaviors. We have emphasized motivated behavioral disorders such as addictions and paraphilias, but it is equally important to consider maladaptive behaviors, such as suicide and self-mutilation, and adaptive behaviors, such as pill taking, when formulating a patient's case. Addictions can be occult, and patients should be evaluated carefully. Addictions may also interfere with the treatment of other problems, but they may actually be a useful tool in the manipulation of patients. Patients addicted to morphine and heroin are nearly universally disordered by their addiction, whereas those addicted to methadone are far less disordered and much more functional. Addiction to methadone brings a patient regularly to a program in which a group drug rehabilitation treatment can be used. It also brings that patient to a clinical setting where depression treatment, HIV care, tuberculosis care, and vocational rehabilitation can occur concurrently. We do not adequately exploit this in our clinic, but some programs have developed this model approach. Additionally, individual clinicians make this work successfully for themselves. They notice that at their monthly visit for chronic pain medications or sedative-hypnotic agents, patients can be successfully "piggybacked" into effective HIV treatment. The risks and benefits of encouraging patients to get detoxified from addictive medications or drugs involves a careful assessment of the degree of disorder the drug is producing, the degree that it is likely to produce with continued use, and the positive utility of the drug.

For patients with other motivated behavior disorders or maladaptive behaviors, interventions that stop such behaviors open the door to the pursuit of new, adaptive behaviors that can easily be applied to the rehabilitative work inherent in any medical illness.

The fourth consideration for all patients is their life circumstances, both the daily circumstance of the present and the past experiences that have shaped their views of the world. Assumptions about the world are based on the experiences people have, but they also shape the experiences people have. Trust issues will remain problematic throughout treatment for a person tragically misused in his or her early life. Circumstances are equally important. Patients with small children and chaotic lives will need some level of planning for treatment based on their circumstances. Economic situations are also important barriers to care and are critical in many formulations. A history of repeated unsuccessful treatments might be explained within the domain of personality, as we have described previously, but it may be equally well explained by the disordered health care system of constantly changing doctors, carved-out mental health care, and the conflict of interest between sickness behavior rewarded by disability payments and the patient role of active participation in rehabilitation to resume normal function. Health care workers need to "walk a mile in the shoes of the patient." Understanding *why* patients are noncompliant is as important as figuring out that they *are* noncompliant.

The development of a comprehensive diagnostic formulation will nearly always make a logical course of treatment obvious. The technical end of treatment is important and a considerable challenge to us, but it is of less significance than the method used to determine the appropriate treatment. The most skilled surgeon performing a complicated operation in which technique is so important, such as a pancreatoduodenojejunectomy (a.k.a. a Whipple procedure), is doing the patient no service if that is not the operation he or she needs. The skill of the clinician is as much in knowing when to operate and which operation to do as in doing the operation. Nobody wants a Whipple unless he or she needs one, not even if John Cameron, the wizard of the Whipple at Johns Hopkins, performs it. Besides his skill, what makes Dr. Cameron one of the world's greatest surgeons is knowing when to do a Whipple and when not to.

The Role of the Doctor

Paul McHugh's distillation of the role of the doctor is more useful than any other definition we have heard. He asserts that the doctor's role consists of three elements. First, the doctor is a possessor of a special knowledge base that is a comprehensive digest of all the information relevant to the care of his or her patients. Second, the doctor is an expert at a special procedure of history taking, examination, and diagnosis, as well as an expert in the application of treatments relevant to those patients. Finally, the doctor is an advocate for the patient.

In this regard, the job of the clinician is to evaluate patients, figure out a formulation as previously mentioned, and develop an appropriate treatment plan. He or she is then required to advocate for the patient to receive the treatment and for the patient to accept the treatment. With regard to the complicated patients, it means the clinician must prescribe change, advocate for change, insist on change, demand change, and expect change. Patients often come to believe that change is not possible, and the clinician must be a therapeutic optimist to counteract this. Patients have never before experienced the circumstances they are facing, causing them to feel demoralized and overwhelmed. The clinician must represent the potential for a new life, a better life, and for change.

Physicians who plan for and expect failure are less vulnerable to disappointment when patients do not succeed. Those physicians often get out of patients only what they expect. In the current health care system, they will be rewarded for their husbandry of resources and their ability to treat patients efficiently. They will seldom see miracles and will discount those they do see. It is easy to see why a therapeutically nihilistic approach is appealing. If you plan for the patient to fail, when failure occurs, the treatment outcome is what was expected. On the other hand, if you strive for success in difficult and hopeless cases, some will feel a sense of failure when patients die. However, those that pursue miracles will test the limits of their skills. They will be sharper, be more skilled, and see more miracles.

Good research suggests that the actual rate of medical miracles is approximately 5 percent. A favorite of these studies involved an effort to show the futility of intensive care in a subgroup of patients in Great Britain. The study showed that you could use an instrument to identify patients at extremely high risk for death, but that a number of patients survived and did well unexpectedly. In the author's words, "Prospectively this study supports the ability to predict the futility of continued intensive care but at the cost of 1 in 20 patients who would survive if care were continued."[1]

A Model Structure for an HIV Clinic

Throughout this book, we propose the commitment of resources to HIV-infected patients to improve outcome and diminish transmission. One question is how to deploy the resources that are committed. We have studied this problem in a variety of ways. Our initial model was to provide psychiatric evaluations to patients in the HIV clinic on site and then to refer patients to appropriate care in the community. In 1989/90, we saw 94 successive evaluations (2 each week) for psychiatric care and referred all patients for treatment. Each of the referred patients had a significant psychiatric disorder and morbidity, and we told each patient what we thought was the most likely diagnosis and why it was important to receive treatment. Nearly all patients (89/94) agreed to be referred for treatment. We checked to see if patients were following up, and in that one-year period not one patient made it to the scheduled follow-up (unpublished observation). We were ultimately able to get many of the patients into treatment, but we found that treatment at other sites for psychiatry did not seem optimal for our patients.

We decided that psychiatric care for HIV-infected patients must be provided on site along with other subspecialty services. This was already the model used at Johns Hopkins for other services, with gastroenterology, ophthalmology, dermatology, nutrition, social work, and almost all other disciplines providing care in the clinic alongside the HIV primary care providers. Despite the fact that all other disciplines were represented, we met an initial reluctance to fund our work and found some colleagues surprised that we would come to the HIV clinic rather than have the patients come to psychiatry.

Once we were established in the clinic, the demand for psychiatric evaluation rapidly became intense, and we surveyed the new patients to see the extent and intensity of psychiatric disorders in patients infected with HIV. The numbers were quite high; more than half of the patients surveyed had a psychiatric disorder other than substance abuse that needed treatment, and three-quarters of the patients had a substance use disorder.

Our model of treatment has evolved to provide psychiatric and substance use disorder treatment on site while collaborating with other specialty psychiatric clinics and allied programs in the area to allow for a broad spectrum of services. These include collaborations with vocational rehabilitation, psychosocial rehabilitation programs, and group-therapy-directed programs directed at specific behaviors (weight management, substance use disorders, paraphilia, and gambling).

At the clinic, the psychiatry notes for a patient are filed within the same charts as the medical notes. This allows for maximum communication between the treatment providers. It also diminishes the tendency for patients to "split" the treatment team and to pursue unhealthy goals using clinic resources. We often add notes to the charts such as "no pain meds without discussion," "no benzo," or "tox screen every visit" to alert both our own team and medical colleagues to important issues regarding some particular patient's care.

In this section and the following one, we outline our ideas for an ideal clinic. Ultimately, our goal is to have an integrated rehabilitation program for combined medical, psychosocial, psychiatric, and rehabilitative care in one setting coordinated by a single team of providers. In this model patients would be assessed at intake by a team that would comprehensively assess their needs and goals for treatment. The initial step would be the assembly of a database and a diagnostic formulation addressing all active medical, psychiatric, and social issues, as well as vocational and housing assessments. Patients would be presented with an incentive-driven treatment plan directed at helping them restore health, function, quality of life, and independence. The social service provision would come about through a case management plan that would require the successful completion of steps within the plan before any movement forward, and each step would have incentives built into it for patient care and independence.

The housing arm would be located near the medical center. It would consist of an apartment complex, a halfway house, a supportive care center with a nursing home unit, and an infirmary with a pharmacy. The complex would be supported by its own shop and facilities management unit. A 12-step program meeting site and multi-denominational chapel would also be located on site. The complex would provide security from dangerous outside elements, such as infiltration by drug dealers, as well as security for patients with special issues, such as patients with dementia who might wander. Living quarters would be staged, so that as patients progressed they could gain more independence.

Initial patients with substance use disorders would live in a halfway facility on campus. They would move toward independence by completing treatment goals as described later. All patients would be required to contribute to the housing complex with a predetermined amount of service hours. Many of these services could be provided through on-site vocational rehabilitation in one of the service shop units and would include painting, grounds maintenance, plumbing and heating, carpentry, electrical, food service, personal care, day care, and medical service. Each unit would use the resources of the facility as well as outside experts from the local community who would act as instructors and employees. Patients would gain an incentive to work as employees either outside or at the complex when they reach an appropriate privilege level. They would then be required to pay "rent," a portion of which would help support them when they left the therapeutic community.

Patients would also be required to meet the requirements of their treatment plans to remain in the community. Family members willing to accept the rules of the community would be able to live on site with patients and be able to directly access services as well. Partners and family members unwilling to participate in the therapeutic community would be able to visit only. Any patient that failed to meet his or her treatment goals (such as sobriety) would have visitors restricted to therapeutic sessions only. Patients would be permitted to leave the community at any time, but they would forfeit any resources and accumulated assets that belonged to the community if they were discharged. They could rejoin as well but would need to reestablish a treatment plan and goals.

On-site treatment would include substance use disorder groups, 12-step meetings, drug toxicology monitoring, an infirmary, and a methadone program. The medical clinic service for HIV care would be located on site and would provide most of the clinical services needed by patients. On-site nursing care would also be provided and, when possible, be staffed by and provide training to residents of the community.

The clinic would be a multidisciplinary treatment site providing local patients with treatment for sexually transmitted diseases (STDs), substance use disorders, and HIV infection. As these are all groups at risk for HIV or for infecting others, the provision of well-directed clinical care would help prevent new infections as well as treat established patients. The major factors known to affect compliance, such as substance use disorders and depression, could all be addressed within the clinic as well. The prevention and treatment of tuberculosis and syphilis would also be accomplished on site.

Geographically, the clinic and community would be in contiguity with a medical center that provides residency education. Resident and faculty primary care clinics would be associated with the clinic, allowing for primary care residents to undergo training in substance use disorders and psychiatric care. Expert obstetric and gynecologic treatment in the clinic would decrease vertical transmissions to babies being born into the community.

Clinic Organization

In an ideal clinic, the structure of patient care would be set up to facilitate behavioral changes. New patients would have the services and structure of the clinic explained to them upon arrival. The goal of organizing behavior and changing dysfunctional behavior patterns would also be explained. Routinely, a patient would begin with an appointment, and anyone who misses his or her appointment would have to wait to be seen on a first-come, first-served basis at the weekly unscheduled (walk-in) clinic, which would typically involve a long and relatively uncomfortable wait to be seen. Patients with appointments with care providers would have minimal waits, but if they missed an appointment without having canceled, they would need to wait at an unscheduled clinic to reestablish an appointment. Patients with habits of missing appointments would be forced to come to an unscheduled clinic that would occur weekly for a period of several visits before they could reestablish coming on an appointment basis. Urgent problems would also be seen in an unscheduled clinic, but a triage process at registration would expedite truly urgent patient problems. This method has the advantage of rewarding and shaping positive behavior for patients who arrive at appointments on time. It also increases clinic efficiency by minimizing missed appointments during which clinicians sit inactive.

Referrals for substance use disorder and psychiatric care would be monitored to see if patients were keeping them. Patients requesting controlled drugs, clinic resources outside of medical care, and social interventions would be required to make their appointments for the treatment of disorders that are likely to interfere with their care, thus rewarding adherence to activities designed to promote health and function with more interventions by the staff, rather than supporting a system in which these interventions are seen as entitlements regardless of behavior. Access to detoxification would be available 24 hours a day but would require a commitment on the part of the patient to cooperate with treatment after the detoxification was completed.

As much as possible, all resources, such as public assistance, prescription assistance, government-supported housing, and other social resources, would be provided through a therapeutic contract with patients to modify their behavior toward improved functioning, quality of life, independence, and health.

Paternalism in Medical Care

The previously outlined approach is paternalistic. It intrudes into life decisions made by patients and places the goals of the treatment team ahead of those stated by the patients. The generally implied view in the medical literature is that paternalism is bad. It often begets apologies and a description as a holdover from an earlier era of medicine. This stance is unsupported by data to suggest that the outcome of paternalism is worse than the outcome of care that places patient autonomy first. Although risk invades a paternalistic setting in the form of a doctor who substitutes personal politics for consideration of the patient's wishes, the system of medical ethics is designed to address the limits of paternalism, beginning in the days of the Hippocratic oath. As professionals in possession of special knowledge and skill, the doctor role must inherently bring some degree of paternalism to the frankly unequal doctor-patient relationship. Paternalism may simply manifest itself in a doctor who has adequate experience to weigh factors beyond the experience of the patient.

Although in many circumstances paternalism would be clearly a violation of the autonomy of patients, the idea of autonomy itself needs careful consideration with regards to vulnerable patients. Impaired people have impaired autonomy. Impairment is a dimension, with some patients profoundly impaired, such as our earlier example of the patient with a delusional belief that he had parasites and needed an amputation of his arm. Others are only mildly impaired, such as patients who wish to leave the hospital against medical advice because they crave a resumption of their drug use. The goal of the doctor is to recognize such impairments and, when they are present, weigh the issue of autonomy with the issue of beneficence, which is simply defined as doing what is in the patient's best interests. Such decisions are tempered by judgment, experience, and thought, but essentially they are often difficult to make and even contentious.

The patient-doctor relationship is derived from the inequality of power between doctor and patient. The doctor lives, and in fact is paid, even if the patient dies. This is an unfair relationship for both the patient and the doctor. Because of this, the ethics of medicine require a doctor to put the patient's best interests ahead of his or her own. Making money, personal desires, and profit are to be strictly excluded from the equation except in the form of the "usual and customary" fee. The relationship focuses on the patient's *best* interests, not the patient's *stated* interests. Patients who want narcotics because they like to be intoxicated might say that their best interests are served by a prescription for opiates (in fact, they would certainly say this).

The matter is further complicated by the pressures brought to bear on medical care decisions by the culture, the administrative structures of medicine, and even the politics of the moment. Issues of resource allocation, finance, and reimbursement all may play a role in how a decision is reached. These pressures influence how doctors respond to decisions.

What is the method a physician can use to make a reasonable decision? We recommend that two considerations be placed ahead of others. One is the goal of treatment. Clinicians must define the treatment goals. Patients may wish to focus entirely on comfort or the relief of distress, but the clinician must also consider goals such as function, longevity, and quality of life. These goals can be discussed with patients and the discussion may even persuade them to change their decisions. Obviously, in some cases, these goals cannot be realized, and the goal of comfort becomes primary. Conflicts arise when the patient is focused on the goal of comfort to the exclusion of treatment that will result in improved health. If a patient needs surgery, the goal of comfort is supervened by the goal of saving the patient's life. Comfort is considered by using pain control during the process, but the process is not pain free.

The second consideration is the ratio of risk to benefit. An uncomfortable detoxification may have risks associated with it, including encountering paternalistic doctors and a temporary loss of autonomy. The risks are substantially offset, however, by the potential benefits of improved autonomy once free from the bonds of addiction, improved health, and a diminished risk of contracting HIV and other infections or of spreading those infections. The vulnerable patient is unable to make a reasonable assessment of these risks. His or her judgment and autonomy is impaired in an important way by illness or addiction. Herein lies the license for paternalism in the doctor-patient relationship.

Does this mean that treatment can and should be forced on all patients? In our opinion, the answer is no. Instead, public awareness must be raised as to how such a decision process is made and advocacy must be widespread for incentives to help patients make good decisions. The availability of social supports contingent on decisions directed at improving function will help patients move forward in treatment instead of oscillating between disability and early stages of recovery. Society currently pays people to be disabled, rather than paying them to get better. As soon as they improve, they are penalized by the loss of payments, and periodically the level of illness they must manifest to be paid increases, with a corresponding decrease in their functionality. Social resources have come to be referred to as "entitlements," and patients have come to feel entitled to them rather than seeing them as a means to gain independence and success. Linking resources through medical systems to a successful engagement in treatment and improved functioning can have a huge effect on the outcome and chronicity of illness. Even those with the most genuine disabilities would benefit from the structure, self-esteem, and social interaction that come from a form of occupation and contribution. People are more likely to build and defend a society if they are part of that society and have a role in it.

Managed Care

Health care is currently provided to patients by physicians and other health care providers and is most often paid for by a variety of third-party payers. The doctor is supposed to work for the patient but is actually paid by a third party. This means that the doctor has an obligation to the patient to provide the best possible care, but a financial incentive to deliver care that satisfies the goals of the payer. This threat to the patient-doctor relationship has been opposed by the long tradition of medical commitment to patient care and the reality that when things go badly, the doctor, not the insurance company, is held liable. Payers complain that providers will provide excessive services to patients if they are reimbursed for any and all treatment provided, and that they will have a financial incentive to do so. In fact, one of the factors in the evolution of the current system is the excessive and exuberant commitment to certain procedures and tests that have been quite clearly misused by some unscrupulous doctors.

In an effort to combat what is felt to be unnecessary spending by doctors, the health care system has developed a variety of management systems. These include directly employing physicians, erecting paperwork or other impediments to the provision of care, refusing to pay for care after it has been delivered, and appointing people to review medical care. All these approaches have effectively rationed care and added to the cost of health care. The apologists for the health care industry say this is necessary for financial responsibility in health care. Over time, health care reviewers have changed the standard of medical care from the old standard, that is, treatment is beneficial and the potential benefits outweigh the risks, to treatment that is termed "medically necessary," essentially meaning the patient will die or come to obvious harm without the treatment.

An example of this problem is that 20 years ago, patients were staying in the hospital too long. Being in the hospital has both risks and potential benefits, and the benefits are outweighed by the risks when patients stay there too long. The risks include being exposed to a harmful infection and drug-resistant bacteria, losing the momentum of your life, becoming more and more deconditioned, and becoming dependent on the hospital for functioning. Studies have documented these risks and that lengthy hospitalizations sometimes include risks that doctors had not considered. Shorter stays have resulted in no clear diminishment of the effectiveness of treating most patients. The problem is that the methods that make it difficult for doctors to keep patients in the hospital for longer periods have prevented longer stays for patients who need and benefit from them. In these instances, the stays are not medically necessary for survival, but they are necessary for recovery and rehabilitation, and may mean the difference between a return to an independent life and permanent disability.

As medical care is rationed, those with difficult-to-treat conditions and limited resources receive less treatment. Chronic mental illness is associated with poor health care. A psychiatrist with a private-pay-based practice in a wealthy suburb can make a far better income than a person committed to the treatment of chronically mentally ill persons in the inner city. This has resulted in the development of community-based mental heath programs that tend to be understaffed and inadequately funded. Thus, the sickest patients receive the least care. A person who is worried about whether or not he or she feels fulfilled by life can spend 50 minutes with a doctor to discuss it, whereas a person with chronic hallucinations and delusions may see a therapist for treatment and see the doctor as infrequently as every 3 months for a 15-minute evaluation of medicine effectiveness and side effects.

Many heath care organizations are also keeping track of outcome as a measurement of the quality of care a patient receives. Comparisons do not consider the complexity or severity of patients' illnesses, only how they do after treatment. This means that one way to improve the outcome is to start with patients who are less sick. This was best demonstrated by a hospital in the state of Pennsylvania, where a large effort was made to decrease the morbidity and mortality of patients undergoing cardiac procedures. The efforts to improve the outcomes by improving clinical care were relatively ineffective, but by selecting patients to receive procedures based on lower severity of their sickness, a robust improvement in outcomes occurred. This was good for the managers, who had less intensive care time and fewer complications for which to pay; good for the hospitals, who had fewer costs associated with each case; and good for the clinicians, who had better results and fewer problems. It was really a problem only if you had a complicated cardiac condition and found you could not receive the care you needed.

Imagine the effect this would have on a "managed" medical clinic provider who is paid based on productivity (the number of patients seen each hour) and who receives a bonus based on outcome (fewer hospital admissions, tests, and complications) and customer satisfaction (surveys of whether the patient was pleased). The clinician has the opportunity to see medically complicated psychiatrically ill and substance-abusing patients. Such patients take longer to evaluate and treat, are likely to require extensive tests and have complications, and are seldom pleased unless they get exactly what they request. When a patient presents requesting narcotics or benzodiazepines, the clinician must decide between two options. The first would be to spend an inordinate amount of time explaining why this would be a bad choice of treatment, thus risking a complaint to customer service. The second choice would be to simply give the patient what he or she wants, making the patient happy, saving time, and perhaps even improving the likelihood of the patient coming to his or her next visit. Unfortunately, this is hardly what medical care directed at health and productivity is about. Patients with psychiatric complications require more time, need more evaluation, and require more services in general.

An essential problem in the HIV epidemic is that quarterly profits have come to drive the management of health care. The companies that pay for health care have no incentive to stop the HIV epidemic. Front-loaded costs spent now to prevent future infections and disease do little to help the immediate bottom line. Money spent on rehabilitation yields no financial benefit to the health care company that reimburses care.

Inadequate attention has been paid to how this approach has shifted resources away from patients, developed enormous profits to companies that do not provide any health care service at all except to restrict it, and deprived the most vulnerable patients of care. Vulnerable (mentally ill, minority, poor, isolated, and disenfranchised) patients have no voice and few advocates. They are carved out of care, and their basic health care issues are ignored.

Although managed care and health maintenance organizations have integrated themselves into the system of care delivery to presumably decrease health care costs, they have been ineffective in decreasing the amount of the gross national product spent on health care. However, they have diverted a substantial part of the finance to huge administrative structures that provide nothing but an obstruction to care.

What will improve health care and decrease the HIV epidemic are financial programs that make health care systems attend to the future costs of care as much as the present ones. Investments in drug treatment prevent crime, arrests, court costs, prison and parole costs, and, most important, the costs of HIV care. Investments in psychiatric treatment improve the financial independence and success of patients and their outcome, and they also improve compliance with antiretroviral care. These are modest costs compared with what we spend on other responses to the epidemic.

During the huge surge of interest in health care reform that helped to drive the first Clinton presidential campaign, the media hammered the public with the figure that the United States was spending 13 percent of the gross national product on health care but ignored the fact that we spend almost one-third of it on entertainment. The expenditures on biomedical research and health care have effectively lengthened the life expectancy of the average person 30 years over what it was in the nineteenth century. The health care industry has also developed four new classes of antiretroviral drugs that were inconceivable 15 years ago. We submit that we have made far more progress with our 13 percent of the GNP than the entertainment industry has with its third.

Summary

Throughout this book, we have suggested that certain patients with the highest risk for contracting and spreading HIV are those who are most vulnerable due to mental illness. The vulnerabilities are treatable and respond to a therapeutically optimistic approach. In this chapter, we have outlined a method by which such optimism can be implemented for patients. Some parts of what we have described are already operational in our clinic and other clinics, but many of the ideas here require a fundamental modification in the way services are delivered and funded. It will be difficult to persuade those who evaluate health care costs on a quarterly basis and who have little incentive for upfront investments to take the ideas here toward implementation. On the other hand, those who are concerned about the HIV epidemic, the hepatitis C epidemic, and the lives and well-being of our patients may find tremendous empowerment in this approach.

Notes

Chapter *1:* Why AIDS Psychiatry?

1. Moreno A, Perez-Elias MJ, Casado JL, Munoz V, Antela A, Dronda F, Navas E, Fortun J, Quereda C, Moreno S. Effectiveness and pitfalls of initial highly active anti-retroviral therapy in HIV-infected patients in routine clinical practice. *Antiviral Therapy* 2000 Dec.;5(4):243–8.

2. Paterson DL, Swindells S, Mohr J, Brester M, Vergis EN, Squier C, Wagener MM, Singh N. Adherence to protease inhibitor therapy and outcomes in patients with HIV infection. *Annals of Internal Medicine* 2000;133:21–30.

3. Singh N, Squier C, Sivek C, Wagener M, Nguyen MH, Yu VL. Determinants of compliance with antiretroviral therapy in patients with human immunodeficiency virus: prospective assessment with implications for enhancing compliance. *AIDS Care* 1996; 8:261–9.

4. Lucas GM, Chaisson RE, Moore RD. Highly active antiretroviral therapy in a large urban clinic: risk factors for virologic failure and adverse drug reactions. *Annals of Internal Medicine* 1999;131:81–7.

5. American Psychiatric Association. *Diagnostic and Statistical Manual of Mental Disorders*, 4th edition. Washington, D.C.: American Psychiatric Association, 1994.

6. Atkinson S, Bihari D, Smithies M, Daly K, Mason R, McColl I. Identification of futility in intensive care. *Lancet* 1994;344:203–6.

7. Zhu T, Korber BT, Nahmias AJ, Hooper E, Sharp PM, Ho DD. An African HIV-1 sequence from 1959 and implications for the origin of the epidemic. *Nature* 1998 Feb. 5;391(6667):594–7.

8. Verghese A. *My Own Country: A Doctor's Story*. New York: Random House, 1995.

9. Treisman G, Fishman M, Lyketsos C, McHugh PR. Evaluation and treatment of psychiatric disorders associated with HIV infection. In Price RW, Perry SW, eds., *HIV, AIDS and the Brain*. New York: Raven Press, 1994.

10. Mellors JW, Rinaldo CR Jr., Gupta P, White RM, Todd JA, Kingsley LA. Prognosis in HIV-1 infection predicted by the quantity of virus in plasma. *Science* 1996;272:1167–70.

11. Ho DD, Neumann AU, Perelson AS, Chen W, Leonard JM, Markowitz M. Rapid turnover of plasma virions and CD4 lymphocytes in HIV-1 infection. *Nature* 1995;373: 123–6.

12. Palella FJ Jr., Delaney KM, Moorman AC, Loveless MO, Fuher J, Satten GA, Aschman DJ, Holmsberg SD. Declining morbidity and mortality among patients with advanced human immunodeficiency virus infection. *New England Journal of Medicine* 1998;338:853–60.

13. Hogg RS, O'Shaughnessy MV, Gataric N, Yip B, Craib K, Schecter MT, Montaner JS. Decline in deaths from AIDS due to new antiretrovirals. *Lancet* 1997;349:1294.

14. Cameron DW, Heath-Chiozzi M, Kravcik S, et al. Prolongation of life and prevention of AIDS complications in advanced HIV immunodeficiency with ritonavir: update [abstract Mo.B.411]. In: Abstracts of the 11th International Conference on AIDS, Vancouver, 1996;1:24.

15. Brenner BG, Wainberg MA. The role of antiretrovirals and drug resistance in vertical transmission of HIV-1 infection. *Annals of the New York Academy of Science* 2000; 918:9–15.

16. Henderson DK. Postexposure chemoprophylaxis for occupational exposures to the human immunodeficiency virus. *JAMA* 1999;281:931–6.

17. Anastos K, Gange SJ, Lau B, Weiser B, Detels R, Giorgi JV, Margolick JB, Cohen M, Phair J, Melnick S, Rinaldo CR, Kovacs A, Levine A, Landesman S, Young M, Munoz A, Greenblatt RM. Association of race and gender with HIV-1 RNA levels and immunologic progression. *Journal of Acquired Immune Deficiency Syndromes* 2000 July; 124(3): 218–26.

18. Carpenter CC, Fischl MA, Hammer SM, Hirsch MS, Jacobsen DM, Katzenstein DA, Montaner JS, Richman DD, Saag MS, Schooley RT, Thompson MA, Vella S, Yeni PG, Volberding PA. Antiretroviral therapy for HIV infection in 1998: Updated recommendations of the International AIDS Society—USA Panel. *JAMA* 1998;280:78–86.

19. McHugh PR, Slavney PR. *The Perspectives of Psychiatry*, 2nd edition. Baltimore: Johns Hopkins University Press, 1998.

Chapter *2:* HIV and Major Depression

1. Dimatteo MR, Lepper HS, Croghan TW. Depression is a risk factor for noncompliance with medical treatment. *Archives of Internal Medicine* 2000;160:2101–7.

2. Lenz G, Demal U. Quality of life in depression and anxiety disorders: An exploratory follow-up after intensive cognitive-behavior therapy. *Psychopathology* 2000; 33:297–302.

3. Meltzer-Brody S, Davidson JR. Completeness of response and quality of life in mood and anxiety disorders. *Depression and Anxiety* 2000;12 Suppl. 1:95–101.

4. Holmes J, House A. Psychiatric illness predicts poor outcome after surgery for hip fracture: a prospective cohort study. *Psychological Medicine* 2000;30:921–9.

5. Orr S, Celentano DD, Santelli J, Burwell L. Depressive symptoms and risk factors for HIV acquisition among black women attending urban health centers in Baltimore. *AIDS Education and Prevention* 1994;6:230–6.

6. Nyamathi A. Comparative study of factors relating to HIV risk level of black homeless women. *Journal of Acquired Immune Deficiency Syndromes* 1992;5:222–8.

7. Morrill AC, Ickovics JR, Golubchikov VV, Beren SE, Rodin J. Safer sex: social and psychological predictors of behavioral maintenance and change among heterosexual women. *Journal of Consulting and Clinical Psychology* 1996;64:819–28.

8. Perkins DO, Leserman J, Stern RA, Baum SF, Liao D, Golden RN, Evans DL. Somatic symptoms and HIV infection: Relationship to depressive symptoms and indicators of HIV disease. *American Journal of Psychiatry* 1995;155(12):1776–81.

9. Pugh K, Riccio M, Jadresic D, Burgess AP, Baldeweg T, Catalan J, Lovett E, Hawkins DA, Gruzelier J, Thompson C. A longitudinal study of the neuropsychiatric consequences of HIV-1 infection in gay men. II Psychological and health status at baseline and at 12-month follow-up. *Psychological Medicine* 1994;24:897–904.

10. Grinspoon S, Corcoran C, Stanley T, Baaj A, Basgoz N, Klibanski A. Effects of hypogonadism and testosterone administration on depression indices in HIV-infected men. *Journal of Clinical Endocrinology and Metabolism* 2000;85:60–5.

11. Lyketsos CG, Hanson A, Fishman M, McHugh PR, Treisman GJ. Screening for psychiatric morbidity in a medical outpatient clinic for HIV infection: the need for a psychiatric presence. *International Journal of Psychiatry in Medicine* 1994;24:103–13.

12. Rabkin JG, Rabkin R, Harrison W, Wagner G. Effects of imipramine on mood and immune status in depressed patients with HIV illness. *American Journal of Psychiatry* 1994;151:516–23.

13. Rabkin JG, Rabkin R, Wagner G. Fluoxetine effects on mood and immune status in depressed patients with HIV illness. *Journal of Clinical Psychiatry* 1994;55:433–9.

14. Rabkin JG, Wagner G, Rabkin R. Sertraline effects on mood and immune status in depressed patients with HIV illness: an open trial. *Journal of Clinical Psychiatry* 1994;55:92–7.

15. Grassi B, Gambini O, Garchentini G, Lazzarin A, Scarone S. Efficacy of paroxetine in the treatment of depression in the context of HIV infection. *Pharmacopsychiatry* 1997;30:70–1.

16. Elliott AJ, Uldall KK, Bergam K, Ruso J, Claypoole K, Roy-Byrne PP. Randomized, placebo-controlled trial of paroxetine versus imipramine in depressed HIV-positive outpatients. *American Journal of Psychiatry* 1998;155:367–72.

17. Rabkin JG, Wagner GJ, Rabkin R. Fluoxetine treatment for depression in patients with HIV and AIDS: a randomized, placebo-controlled trial. *American Journal of Psychiatry* 1999;156:101–7.

18. Schwartz JAJ, McDaniel S. Double-blind comparison of fluoxetine and desipramine in the treatment of depressed women with advanced HIV disease: a pilot study. *Depression and Anxiety* 1999;9:70–4.

19. Fernandez F, Levy JK, Samley HR, Pirozzolo FJ, Lachar D, Crowley J, Adams S, Ross B, Ruiz P. Effects of methylphenidate in HIV-related depression: a comparative trial with desipramine. *International Journal of Psychiatry in Medicine* 1995;25:53–67.

20. Wagner GJ, Rabkin JG, Rabkin R. A comparative analysis of standard and alternative antidepressants in the treatment of human immunodeficiency virus patients. *Comprehensive Psychiatry* 1996;37:402–8.

21. Elliott AJ, Roy-Byrne PP. Major depressive disorder and HIV-1 infection: a review of treatment trials. *Seminars in Clinical Neuropsychiatry* 1998;3:137–50.

22. Glassman AH, Perel JM, Shostak M, Kantor KJ, Fleiss JL. Clinical implications of imipramine plasma levels for depressive illness. *Archives of General Psychiatry* 1977;34:197–204.

23. Asberg M, Cronholm B, Sjoqvist F, Tuck D. Relationship between plasma level and therapeutic effect of nortriptyline. *British Medical Journal* 1971;3:331–4.

24. Ziegler VE, Clayton PJ, Taylor JR, Tee B, Biggs JT. Nortriptyline plasma levels and therapeutic response. *Clinical Pharmacology and Therapeutics* 1976;20:458–63.

25. Rothschild AJ. New directions in the treatment of antidepressant-induced sexual dysfunction. *Clinical Therapeutics* 2000;22 Suppl. A:A42–A51; discussion A58–A61.

26. Woodrum ST, Brown CS. Management of SSRI-induced sexual dysfunction. *Annals of Pharmacotherapy* 1998;32:1209–15.

27. Heninger GR, Charney DS, Sternberg DE. Lithium carbonate augmentation of antidepressant treatment: An effective prescription for treatment refractory depression. *Archives of General Psychiatry* 1983;40:1335–42.

28. Neirenberg AA, Price LH, Charney DS, Heninger GR. After lithium augmentation: A retrospective follow-up of patients with antidepressant-refractory depression. *Journal of Affective Disorders* 1990;18:167–75.

29. Stein G, Bernadt M. Lithium augmentation therapy in tricyclic-resistant depression: A controlled trial using lithium in low and normal doses. *British Journal of Psychiatry* 1993;162:634–40.

30. Katona CLE, Abou-Saleh MT, Harrison DA, Nairac BA, Edwards DR, Lock T, Burns RA, Robertson MM. Placebo-controlled trial of lithium augmentation of fluoxetine and lofepramine. *British Journal of Psychiatry* 1995;166:80–6.

31. Ogura C, Okuma T, Uchida Y, Imai S, Yogi H. Combined thyroid (triiodothyronine)-tricyclic antidepressant treatment in depressed states. *Folia Psychiatrica Neurologica Japonica* 1974;28:179–86.

32. Joffe RT, Levitt AJ, Bagby M, MacDonald C, Singer W. Predictors of response to lithium and triiodothyronine augmentation of antidepressants in tricyclic non-responders. *British Journal of Psychiatry* 1993;163:574–8.

33. Shelton RC, Tollefson GD, Tohen M, Stahl S, Gannon KS, Jacobs TG, Buras WR, Bymaster FP, Zhang W, Spencer KA, Feldman PD, Meltzer HY. A novel augmentation strategy for treating resistant major depression. *American Journal of Psychiatry* 2001; 158:131–4.

34. Papkostas GI, Petersen TJ, Nierenberg AA, Murakami JL, Alpert JE, Rosenbaum JF, Fava M. Ziprasidone augmentation of selective serotonin reuptake inhibitors (SSRIs) for SSRI-resistant major depressive disorder. *Journal of Clinical Psychiatry* 2004;65:217–21.

35. Thase ME, Blomgren SL, Birkett MA, Apter JT, Tepner RG. Fluoxetine treatment of patients with major depressive disorder who failed initial treatment with sertraline. *Journal of Clinical Psychiatry* 1997;58:16–21.

36. Keller MB, McCullough JP, Klein DN, Arnow B, Dunner DL, Gelenberg AJ, Markowitz JC, Nemeroff CB, Russell JM, Thase ME, Trivedi MH, Zajecka J. A comparison of nefazodone, the cognitive behavioral-analysis system of psychotherapy, and their combination for the treatment of chronic depression. *New England Journal of Medicine* 2000;342:1462–70.

37. Frank JD, Frank JB. *Persuasion and Healing: A Comparative Study of Psychotherapy*, 3rd edition. Baltimore: Johns Hopkins University Press, 1991.

38. Markowitz JC, Kocsis JH, Fishman B, Spielman LA, Jacobsberg LB, Frances AJ, Klerman GL, Perry SW. Treatment of depressive symptoms in human immunodeficiency virus-positive patients. *Archives of General Psychiatry* 1998;55:452–7.

39. Kelly JA, Murphy DA, Bahr GR, Kalichman SC, Morgan MG, Stevenson LY, Koob JJ, Brasfield TL, Bernstein BM. Outcome of cognitive-behavioral and support group brief therapies for depressed, HIV-infected persons. *American Journal of Psychiatry* 1993;150: 1679–86.

40. Lee MR, Cohen L, Hadley SW, Godwin FK. Cognitive-behavioral group therapy with medication for depressed gay men with AIDS or symptomatic HIV infection. *Psychiatric Services* 1999;50:948–52.

Chapter *3:* Other Psychiatric Diseases in the HIV Clinic

1. Inouye SK, Charpentier PA. Precipitating factors for delirium in hospitalized elderly persons: predictive model and interrelationship with baseline vulnerability. *JAMA* 1996;275:852–7.

2. Tune L, Carr S, Hoag E, Cooper T. Anticholinergic effects of drugs commonly prescribed for the elderly: potential means for assessing risk of delirium. *American Journal of Psychiatry* 1992;149:1393–4.

3. Navia BA, Cho ES, Petiio CK, Price RW. The AIDS dementia complex: II Neuropathology. *Annals of Neurology* 1986;19:525–35.

4. Reyes MG, Faraldi F, Senseng CS, Flowers C, Fariello R. Nigral degeneration in acquired immune deficiency syndrome (AIDS). *Acta Neuropathologica* 1991;82:39–44.

5. Van Gorp WG, Miller EN, Satz P, Visscher B. Neuropsychological performance in HIV-1-immunocompromised patients: a preliminary report. *Journal of Clinical and Experimental Neuropsychology* 1989;11:763–73.

6. Hestad K, McArthur JH, Dal Pan GJ, Selnes OA, Nance-Sproson TE, Aylward E, Matthews VP, McArthur JC. Regional brain atrophy in HIV-1 infection: association with specific neuropsychological test performance. *Acta Neurologica Scandinavica* 1993;88:112–8.

7. Koutsilieri E, Sopper S, Scheller C, ter Meulen V, Riederer P. Parkinsonism in HIV dementia. *Journal of Neural Transmission* 2002;109:767–75.

8. Hriso E, Kuhn T, Masdeu JC, Grundman M. Extrapyramidal symptoms due to dopamine-blocking agents in patients with AIDS encephalopathy. *American Journal of Psychiatry* 1991;148:1558–61.

9. Maggi P, de Mari M, Moramarco A, Fiorentino G, Lamberti P, Angarano G. Parkinsonism in a patient with AIDS and cerebral opportunistic granulomatous lesions. *Neurological Sciences* 2000;21:173–6.

10. Power C, Selnes O, Grim JA, McArthur JC. The HIV-dementia scale: a rapid screening test. *Journal of Acquired Immune Deficiency Syndromes and Human Retrovirology* 1995;8:273–8.

11. Dougherty RH, Skolasky MA Jr., McArthur JC. Progression of HIV-associated dementia treated with HAART. *AIDS Reader* 2002;69–74.

12. Mijch AM, Judd FK, Lyketsos CG, Ellen S, Cockram SA. Seconday mania in patients with HIV infection: Are antiretrovirals protective? *Journal of Neuropsychiatry and Clinical Neuroscience* 1999;11:475–80.

13. Dunlop O, Bjørklund R, Bruun JN, Evensen R, Goplen AK, Liestøl K, Sannes M, Mæhlen J, Myrvang B. Early psychomotor slowing predicts the development of HIV dementia and autopsy-verified HIV encephalitis. *Acta Neurologica Scandinavica* 2002;105:270–5.

14. Glass JD, Fedor H, Wesselingh SL, McArthur JC. Immunocytochemical quantitation of HIV in the brain: correlation with HIV-associated dementia. *Annals of Neurology* 1995;38:755–62.

15. Portegies P. *The Neurology of HIV-1 Infection*. London: MediTech Media, 1995.

16. Brenneman DE, Westbrook GL, Fitzgerald SP, Ennist DL, Elkins KL, Ruff MR, Pert CB. Neuronal cell killing by the envelope protein of HIV and its prevention by vasoactive intestinal peptide. *Nature* 1988;335:639–42.

17. Lipton SA, Sucher NJ, Kaiser PK, Dreyer EB. Synergistic effects of HIV coat protein and NMDA-receptor medicated neurotoxicity. *Neuron* 1991;7:111–8.

18. Sacktor N, Lyles RH, Skolasky R, Kleeberger C, Selnes OA, Miller EN, Becker JT, Cohen B, McArthur JC, and the Multicenter AIDS Cohort Study. HIV-associated neurologic disease incidence changes: Multicenter AIDS Cohort Study, 1990–1998. *Neurology* 2001;56:257–60.

19. Brodt HR, Kamps BS, Gute P, Knupp B, Staszevski S, Helm EB. Changing incidence of AIDS-defining illnesses in the era of antiretroviral combination therapy. *AIDS* 1997;11:1731–8.

20. Thurnher, MM, Schindler EG, Thurnher SA, Pernerstorfer-Schön H, Kleibl-Popov C, Rieger A. Highly active antiretroviral therapy for patients with AIDS dementia complex: effect on MR imaging findings and clinical course. *American Journal of Neuroradiology* 2000;21:670–8.

21. Kure K, Weidenheim KM, Lyman WD, Dickson DW. Morphology and distribution of HIV-1 gp41-positive microglia in subacute AIDS encephalitis. Pattern of involvement resembling a multisystem degeneration. *Acta Neuropathologica* (Berlin) 1990;80: 393–400.

22. Brew BJ, Rosemblum M, Cronin K, Price RW. AIDS dementia complex and HIV-1 brain infection: clinical-virological correlations. *Annals of Neurology* 1995;38:563–70.

23. Chang L, Speck O, Miller E, Braun J, Jovicich J, Koch C, Itti L, Ernst T. Neural correlates of attention and working memory deficits in HIV patients. *Neurology* 2001;57: 1001–7.

24. Ernst T, Chang L, Jovicich J, Ames N, Arnold S. Abnormal brain activation on functional MRI in cognitively asymptomatic HIV patients. *Neurology* 2002;59:1343–9.

25. Fischl MA, Daikos GL, Uttamchandani RB, Richman DD, Grieco MH, Gottleib MS, Volberding PA, Laskin OL, Leedom JM, Groopman JE, Mildvan D, Schooley RT, Jackson GJ, Durack DT, King D, and the AZT Collaborative Working Group. The efficacy of azidothymidine (AZT) in the treatment of patients with AIDS and AIDS-related complex. *New England Journal of Medicine* 1987;317:185–91.

26. Sacktor NC, Skolasky RL, Lyles RH, Esposito D, Selnes OA, McArthur JC. Improvement in HIV-associated motor slowing after antiretroviral therapy including protease inhibitors. *Journal of Neurovirology* 2000;6:84–8.

27. Dougherty RH, Skolasky RL Jr., McArthur JC. Progression of HIV-associated dementia treated with HAART. *AIDS Reader* 2002;12:69–74.

28. Husstedt IW, Frohne L, Bockenholt S, Frese A, Rahmann A, Heese C, Reichelt D, Evers S. Impact of highly active antiretroviral therapy on cognitive processing in HIV infection: cross-sectional and longitudinal studies of event-related potentials. *AIDS Research and Human Retroviruses* 2002;18:485–90.

29. Chang L, Ernst T, Leonido-Yee M, Witt M, Speck O, Walot I, Miller EN. Highly active antiretroviral therapy reverses brain metabolite abnormalities in mild HIV dementia. *Neurology* 1999;53:782–9.

30. Chang L, Witt M, Eric M, et al. Cerebral metabolite changes during the first nine months after HAART. Abstract S63.001. American Academy of Neurology, May 11, 2001. Philadelphia.

31. Gendelman HE, Zheng J, Coulter CL, Ghorpade A, Che M, Thylin M, Rubocki R, Persidsky Y, Hahn F, Reinhard J Jr., Swindells S. Suppression of inflammatory neurotoxins by highly active antiretroviral therapy in human immunodeficiency virus-associated dementia. *Journal of Infectious Disease* 1998;178:1000–7.

32. Brown GR. The use of methyphenidate for cognitive decline associated with HIV disease. *International Journal of Psychiatry in Medicine* 1995;25:21–37.

33. Chatterjee A, Fahn S. Methylphenidate treats apathy in Parkinson's disease. *Journal of Neuropsychiatry and Clinical Neuroscience* 2002;14:461–2.

34. Forstein M, personal communication, October, 2002.

35. Visscher PM, Yazdi MH, Jackson AD, Schalling M, Lindblad K, Yuan QP, Porteous D, Muir WJ, Blackwood DH. Genetic survival analysis of age-at-onset of bipolar disorder: evidence for anticipation or cohort effect in families. *Psychiatric Genetics* 2001;11:129–37.

36. Jones I, Gordon-Smith K, Craddock N. Triplet repeats and bipolar disorder. *Current Psychiatry Reports* 2002;4:134–40.

37. Ghaemi SN, Boiman EE, Goodwin FK. Kindling and second messengers: an approach to the neurobiology of recurrence in bipolar disorder. *Biological Psychiatry* 1999;45:137–44.

38. Kiburtz K, Zettelmaier AE, Ketonen L, Tuite M, Caine EC. Manic syndrome in AIDS. *American Journal of Psychiatry* 1991;148:1068–70.

39. Lyketsos CG, Schwartz J, Fishman M, Treisman G. AIDS mania. *Journal of Neuropsychiatry and Clinical Neuroscience* 1997;9:277–9.

40. Lyketsos CG, Hanson AL, Fishman M, Rosenblatt A, McHugh PR, Treisman GJ. Manic syndrome early and late in the course of HIV. *American Journal of Psychiatry* 1993;150:326–7.

41. McKinnon K, Cournos F, Sugden R, Guido JR, Herman R. The relative contributions of psychiatric symptoms and AIDS knowledge to HIV risk behaviors among people with severe mental illness. *Journal of Clinical Psychiatry* 1996;57:506–13.

42. Kelly J, Murphy D, Bahr R, Brasfield T, Davis D, Hauth A, Morgan M, Stevenson Y, Eilers K. AIDS/HIV risk behavior among the chronic mentally ill. *American Journal of Psychiatry* 1992;149:886–9.

43. Cournos F, Guido JR, Coomaraswamy S, Meyer-Bahlburg H, Sugden R, Horwath E. Sexual activity and risk of HIV infection among patients with schizophrenia. *American Journal of Psychiatry* 1994;151:228–32.

44. Coverdale JH, Turbott SH, Roberts H. Family planning needs and STD risk behaviours of female psychiatric out-patients. *British Journal of Psychiatry* 1997;171:69–72.

45. Volavka J, Convit A, O'Donnell J, Douyon R, Evangelista C, Czobor P. Assessment of risk behaviors for HIV infection among psychiatric inpatients. *Hospital and Community Psychiatry* 1992;43:482–5.

46. Cournos F, Empfield M, Horwath E, McKinnon K, Meyer I, Schrage H, Currie C, Agosin B. HIV seroprevalence among patients admitted to two psychiatric hospitals. *American Journal of Psychiatry* 1991;148:1225–30.

47. Empfield M, Cournos F, Meyer I, McKinnon K, Horwath E, Silver M, Schrage H, Herman R. HIV seroprevalence among homeless patients admitted to a psychiatric inpatient unit. *American Journal of Psychiatry* 1993;150:47–52.

48. Meyer I, McKinnon K, Cournos F, Empfield M, Bavli S, Engel D, Weinstock A. HIV seroprevalence among long-stay patients in a state psychiatric hospital. *Hospital and Community Psychiatry* 1993;44:282–4.

49. Susser E, Valencia E, Conover S. Prevalence of HIV infection among psychiatric patients in a New York City men's shelter. *American Journal of Public Health* 1993;83: 568–70.

50. Rosenberg SD, Goodman LA, Osher FC, Swartz MS, Essock SM, Butterfield MI, Constantine NT, Wolford GL, Salyers MP. Prevalence of HIV, hepatitis B, and hepatitis C in people with severe mental illness. *American Journal of Gastroenterology* 2001;91:31–7.

51. Katz RC, Watts C, Santman J. AIDS knowledge and high risk behaviors in the chronic mentally ill. *Community Mental Health Journal* 1994;30:395–402.

52. Aruffo JF, Coverdale JH, Chacko RC. Knowledge about AIDS among women psychiatric outpatients. *Hospital and Community Psychiatry* 1990;41:326–8.

53. Zafrani M, McLaughlin DG. Knowledge about AIDS (letter). *Hospital and Community Psychiatry* 1990;41:1261.

54. McDermott BE, Sautter FJ, Winstead DK, Quirk T. Diagnosis, health beliefs, and risk of HIV infection in psychiatric patients. *Hospital and Community Psychiatry* 1994;45: 580–5.

55. Chuang HT, Atkinson M. AIDS knowledge and high-risk behaviour in the chronic mentally ill. *Canadian Journal of Psychiatry* 1996;41:269–72.

56. Akhtar S, Thompson JA. Schizophrenia and sexuality: A report of twelve unusual cases, part II. *Journal of Clinical Psychiatry* 1980;41:166–74.

57. Lukianowicz N. Sexual drive and its gratification in schizophrenia. *International Journal of Social Psychiatry* 1963;9:250–8.

58. Klaf FS, Davis CA. Homosexuality and paranoid schizophrenia: A survey of 150 cases and controls. *American Journal of Psychiatry* 1960;116:1070–5.

59. Lyketsos GC, Sakka P, Mailis A. The sexual adjustment of chronic schizophrenics: a preliminary study. *British Journal of Psychiatry* 1983;143:376–82.

60. McDermott BE, Sautter FJ, Winstead DK, Quirk T. Diagnosis, health beliefs, and risk of HIV infection in psychiatric patients. *Hospital and Community Psychiatry* 1994;45: 580–5.

61. Gewirtz G, Horwath E, Cournos F, Empfield M. Patients at risk for HIV. *Hospital and Community Psychiatry* 1988;39:1311–2.

62. Cournos F, McKinnon K, Mayer-Bahlburg H, Guido JR, Meyer I. HIV risk activity among persons with severe mental illness: preliminary findings. *Hospital and Community Psychiatry* 1993;44:1104–6.

63. Sitzman BT, Burch EA, Bartlett LS, Urrutia G. Rates of sexually transmitted diseases among patients in a psychiatric emergency service. *Psychiatric Services* 1995;46: 136–40.

64. Kelly JA, Murphy DA, Sikkema KJ, Somlai AM, Mulry GW, Fernandez MI, Miller JG, Stevenson LY. Predictors of high and low levels of HIV risk behavior among adults with chronic mental illness. *Psychiatric Services* 1995;46:813–8.

65. Miller LJ, Finnerty M. Sexuality, pregnancy, and childrearing among women with schizophrenia-spectrum disorders. *Psychiatric Services* 1996;47:502–6.

66. Kalichman SC, Kelly JA, Johnson JR, Bulto M. Factors associated with risk for HIV infection among chronic mentally ill patients. *American Journal of Psychiatry* 1994;151:221–7.

67. Baer JW, Dwyer PC, Lewitter-Koehler S. Knowledge about AIDS among psychiatric inpatients. *Hospital and Community Psychiatry* 1988;39:986–8.

68. Jacobs P, Bobek SC. Sexual needs of the schizophrenic client. *Perspectives in Psychiatric Care* 1991;27:15–20.

69. Carmen E, Brady SM. AIDS risk and prevention in the chronic mentally ill. *Hospital and Community Psychiatry* 1990;41:652–7.

70. Kalichman SC, Sikkema KJ, Kelly JA, Bulto M. Use of a brief behavioral skills intervention to prevent HIV infection among chronic mentally ill adults. *Psychiatric Services* 1995;46:275–80.

71. Goisman RM, Kent AB, Montgomery EC, Cheevers MM, Goldfinger SM. AIDS education for patients with chronic mental illness. *Community Mental Health Journal* 1991;27:189–97.

72. Schneier FR, Siris SG. A review of psychoactive substance use and abuse in schizophrenia patterns of drug choice. *Journal of Nervous and Mental Disease* 1987;175: 641–52.

73. Miller FT, Tanenbaum JH. Drug abuse in schizophrenia. *Hospital and Community Psychiatry* 1989;40:847–9.

74. Drake RE, Wallach MA. Substance abuse among the chronic mentally ill. *Hospital and Community Psychiatry* 1989;40:1041–6.

75. Test MA, Wallisch LS, Allness DJ, Ripp K. Substance use in young adults with schizophrenic disorders. *Schizophrenia Bulletin* 1989;15:465–76.

76. Caton CLM, Gralnick A, Bender S, Robert S. Young chronic patients and substance. *Hospital and Community Psychiatry* 1989;40:1037–40.

77. Drake RE, Osher FC, Wallachal A. Alcohol use in abuse in schizophrenia. *Journal of Nervous and Mental Disease* 1989;177:408–14.

78. Mueser KT, Yarnold PR, Levinson DF, Singh H, Bellack AS, Kee K, Morrison RL, Yadalam KG. Revalence of substance abuse in schizophrenia: demographic and clinical correlates. *Schizophrenia Bulletin* 1990;16:31–49.

79. Dixon L, Hass G, Weiden PJ, Sweeney J, Frances AJ. Drug abuse in schizophrenic patients: clinical correlates and reasons for use. *American Journal Psychiatry* 1991;148: 224–30.

80. Mueser KT, Bellack AS, Blanchard JJ. Comorbidity of schizophrenia and substance abuse: implications for treatment. *Journal of Consulting and Clinical Psychology* 1992;60: 845–56.

81. Toner BB, Gillies LA, Prendergast P, Cote FH, Browne C. Substance use disorders in a sample of Canadian patients with chronic mental illness. *Hospital and Community Psychiatry* 1992;43:251–4.

82. Horwath E, Cournos F, McKinnon K, Guido JR, Herman R. Illicit-drug injection among psychiatric patients without a primary substance use disorder. *Psychiatric Services* 1996;47:181–5.

83. Drake RE, Mueser KT, Clark RE, Wallach MA. The course, treatment, and outcome of substance disorder in persons with severe mental illness. American Orthopsychiatric Association, Inc. 1996;66:42–51.

84. Lamb HR. Young adult chronic patients: the new drifters. *Hospital and Community Psychiatry* 1982;197–203.

85. Dixon L, Hass G, Weiden PJ, Sweeney J, Frances AJ. Drug abuse in schizophrenic patients: clinical correlates and reasons for use. *American Journal of Psychiatry* 1991;148:224–30.

86. Alterman AI, Erdlen FR, LaPorte DJ. Effects of illicit drug use in an inpatient psychiatric population. *Addictive Behaviors* 1982;7:231–42.

87. Negrete JC, Knapp WP, Douglas DE. Cannabis affects the severity of schizophrenic symptoms: results of a clinical survey. *Psychological Medicine* 1986;16:515–20.

Chapter *4:* Personality in the HIV Clinic

1. Livesley WJ, Schroeder ML, Jackson DN, Jang K. Categorical distinctions in the study of personality disorder: implication for classification. *Journal of Abnormal Psychology* 1994;103:6–17.

2. Rothbart MK, Ahadi SA. Temperament and the development of personality. *Journal of Abnormal Psychology* 1994;103:55–66.

3. Rutter M. Temperament, personality and personality disorder. *British Journal of Psychiatry* 1987;150:443–58.

4. Jung C. *Personality Types*. Princeton, NJ: Princeton University Press, 1923.

5. Costa PT Jr., Widiger TA, eds. *Personality Disorders and the Five-factor Model of Personality.* Washington, D.C.: American Psychological Association, 1994.

6. Eysenck HJ. Genetic and environmental contributions to individual differences: the three major dimension of personality. *Journal of Personality* 1990;58:245–61.

7. McHugh PR, Slavney PR. *The Perspectives of Psychiatry*, 2nd edition. Baltimore: Johns Hopkins University Press, 1998.

8. Treisman G, Fishman M, Lyketsos C, McHugh PR. Evaluation and treatment of psychiatric disorders associated with HIV infection. In Price RW, Perry SW (eds.), *HIV, AIDS and the Brain.* New York: Raven Press, 1994, pp. 241–50.

9. Eysenck HJ, Rachman S. *The Causes and Cures of Neurosis.* San Diego; Robert R. Knapp, 1965.

10. Eysenck HJ, Eysenck SBG. *Eysenck Personality Questionnaire.* San Diego: EditTS/Educational and Industrial Testing Service, 1975.

11. Eysenck HJ. *Readings in Extraversion-Introversion* (3 vols). New York: Wiley-Interscience, 1970.

12. Eysenck HJ. *Sex and Personality.* London: Open Books, 1976.

13. McCown W. Contributions of the EPN paradigm to HIV prevention: a preliminary study. *Personality and Individual Differences* 1991;12:1301–3.

14. McCown W. Personality factors predicting failure to practice safer sex by HIV-positive males. *Personality and Individual Differences* 1993;14:613–15.

15. Fontaine KL. Unlocking sexual issues. Counseling strategies for nurses. *Nursing Clinics of North America* 1991;26:737–43.

16. Lodhi PH, Thakur S. Personality of drug addicts: Eysenckian analysis. *Personality and Individual Differences* 1993;15:121–8.

17. Francis LJ, Bennett GA. Personality and religion among female drug misusers. *Drug and Alcohol Dependence* 1992;27–31.

18. Francis LJ, Bennett GA. Personality and religion among female drug misusers. *Drug and Alcohol Dependence* 1992;27–31.

19. Paris J. *Social Factors in the Personality Disorders: A Biopsychosocial Approach to Etiology and Treatment.* Cambridge: Cambridge University Press, 1996.

20. Rutter M. Temperament, personality and personality disorder. *British Journal of Psychiatry* 1987;150:443–58.

21. Tourian K, Alterman A, Metzger D, Rutherford M, Cacciola JS, McKay JR. Validity of three measures of antisociality in predicting HIV risk behaviors in methadone-maintenance patients. *Drug and Alcohol Dependence* 1997;47:99–107.

22. Weissman MM. The epidemiology of personality disorders: a 1990 update. *Journal of Personality Disorders* 1993;7(suppl):44–62.

23. Jacobsberg L, Frances A, Perry S. Axis II diagnoses among volunteers for HIV testing and counseling. *American Journal of Psychiatry* 1995;152:1222–4.

24. Johnson JG, Williams JB, Rabkin JG, Goetz RR, Remien RH. Axis I psychiatric symptomatology associated with HIV infection and personality disorder. *American Journal of Psychiatry* 1995;152:551–4.

25. Perkins DO, Davidson EJ, Leserman J, Liao D, Evans DL. Personality disorder in patients infected with HIV: a controlled study with implications for clinical care. *American Journal of Psychiatry* 1993;150:309–15.

26. Golding M, Perkins DO. Personality disorder in HIV infection. *International Reviews in Psychiatry* 1996;8:253–8.

27. American Psychiatric Association. *Diagnostic and Statistical Manual of Mental Disorders*, 4th edition. Washington, D.C.: American Psychiatric Press, 1994.

28. Dinwiddie SH, Cottler L, Compton W, Ben Aabdallah A. Psychopathology and HIV risk behaviors among injection drug users in and out of treatment. *Drug and Alcohol Dependence* 1996;43:1–11.

29. Hudgins R, McCusker J, Stoddard A. Cocaine use and risky injection and sexual behaviors. *Drug and Alcohol Dependence* 1995;37:7–14.

30. Brooner RK, Greenfield L, Schmidt, CW, Bigelow GE. Antisocial personality disorder and HIV infection among intravenous drug users. *American Journal of Psychiatry* 1993;150:53–8.

31. Khantzian EJ, Treece C. DSM-III psychiatric diagnosis of narcotic addicts. *Archives of General Psychiatry* 1985; 42:1067–71.

32. Brooner RK, Bigelow GE, Strian E, Schmidt CW. Intravenous drug users with antisocial personality disorder: increased HIV risk behavior. *Drug and Alcohol Dependence* 1990;26:39–44.

33. Kleinman PH, Millman RB, Robinson H, Lesser M, Hsu C, Engelhart P, Finkelstein I. Lifetime needle sharing: a predictive analysis. *Journal of Substance Abuse and Treatment* 1994;11:449–55.

34. Sackett DL, Snow JS. The magnitude of compliance and noncompliance. In Haynes RB, Taylor DW, Sackett DI, eds., *Compliance in Health Care*. Baltimore: Johns Hopkins University Press, 1979, pp. 11–22.

35. Haynes RB. Determinants of compliance: the disease and the mechanics of treatment. In Haynes RB, Taylor DW, Sackett DI, eds., *Compliance in Health Care*. Baltimore: Johns Hopkins University Press, 1979, pp. 46–62.

36. Blackwell B. From compliance to alliance: a quarter century of research. *Netherlands Journal of Medicine* 1996;48:140–9.

37. Kruse W, Eggert-Kruse W, Rampmaier J, Runnebaum B, Weber E. Dosage frequency and drug-compliance behavior: a comparative study on compliance with a medication to be take twice or four times daily. *European Journal of Clinical Pharmacology* 1991;41d:589–92.

38. Malow RM, McPherson S, Klimas N, Antoni MH, Schneiderman N, Pendo FJ, Ziskind D, Page B, McMahon R, McPherson S. Adherence to complex combination antiretroviral therapies by HIV-positive drug abuser. *Psychiatric Services* 1998;49:1021–2.

39. Eldred LJ, Wu AW, Chaisson RE, Moore RD. Adherence to antiretroviral and pneumocystis prophylaxis in HIV disease. *Journal of AIDS and Human Retroviruses* 1998;18:117–25.

40. Sydenham T. Dissertation epistolaris. 1682, 439n.9.

41. Tanner WM, Pollack RH. The effect of condom use and erotic instructions on attitudes towards condoms. *Journal of Sexual Research* 1988;25:537–41.

42. Abramson PR, Pinkerton SD. *With Pleasure: Thoughts on the Nature of Human Sexuality*. New York: Oxford University Press, 1995.

Chapter 5: Substance Abuse and HIV

1. McHugh PR, Slavney PR. *The Perspectives of Psychiatry*, 2nd edition. Baltimore: Johns Hopkins University Press, 1998.

2. American Psychiatric Association. *Diagnostic and Statistical Manual of Mental Disorders*, 4th edition. Washington, D.C.: American Psychiatric Association, 1994.

3. Prochaska JO, DiClemente CC, Norcross JC. In search of how people change. Applications to addictive behaviors. *American Psychologist* 1997;47:1102–14.

4. Miller WR, Rollnick S. *Motivational Interviewing: Preparing People to Change Addictive Behavior*. New York; Guilford Press, 1991.

Chapter 6: Sexual Problems and HIV

1. Di Giovanni C Jr., Berlin F, Casterella P, Redfield RR, Hiken M, Falck A, Malin HM, Gagliano S, Schaerf F, Roberts C. Prevalence of HIV antibody among a group of paraphilic sex offenders. *Journal of Acquired Immune Deficiency Syndromes* 1991;4(6):633–7.

2. Varella D, Tuason L, Proffitt MR, Escaleira N, Alquezar A, Bukowski RM. HIV infection among Brazilian transvestites in a prison population. *AIDS Patient Care and STDs* 1996 Oct.;10(5):299–302.

3. Nemoto T, Luke D, Mamo L, Ching A, Patria J. HIV risk behaviours among male-to-female transgenders in comparison with homosexual or bisexual males and heterosexual females. *AIDS Care* 1999 June;11(3):297–312.

4. Lubis I, Master J, Munif A, Iskandar N, Bambang M, Papilaya A, Roesin R, Manurung S, Graham R. Second report of AIDS related attitudes and sexual practices of the Jakarta Waria (male transvestites) in 1995. *Southeast Asian Journal of Tropical Medicine and Public Health* 1997 Sept.;28(3):525–9.

5. Gattari P, Speziale D, Grillo R, Cattani P, Zaccarelli M, Spizzichino L, Valenzi C. Syphilis serology among transvestite prostitutes attending an HIV unit in Rome, Italy. *European Journal of Epidemiology* 1994 Dec.;10(6):683–6.

6. Boles J, Elifson KW. The social organization of transvestite prostitution and AIDS. *Social Science in Medicine* 1994 July;39(1):85–93.

7. Elifson KW, Boles J, Posey E, Sweat M, Darrow W, Elsea W. Male transvestite prostitutes and HIV risk. *American Journal of Public Health* 1993 Feb.;83(2):260–2.

8. Clements-Nolle K, Marx R, Guzman R, Katz M. HIV prevalence, risk behaviors, health care use, and mental health status of transgender persons: implications for public health intervention. *American Journal of Public Health* 2001 June;91(6):915–21.

9. Rabkin JG, Wagner GJ, Rabkin R. A double-blind, placebo-controlled trial of testosterone therapy for HIV-positive men with hypogonadal symptoms. *Archives of General Psychiatry* 2000 Feb.;57(2):141–7.

Chapter 7: Life Story Problems in the HIV Clinic

1. Frank JD, Frank JB. *Persuasion and Healing: A Comparative Study of Psychotherapy*, 3rd ed. Baltimore: Johns Hopkins University Press, 1991.

2. Kübler-Ross E. *On Death and Dying.* New York: Macmillan, 1969.

3. Fromm-Reichmann F. Notes on the development of treatment of schizophrenics by psychoanalysis and psychotherapy. *Psychiatry* 1948; 1:263–73.

4. Breslau N. The epidemiology of posttraumatic stress disorder: what is the extent of the problem? *Journal of Clinical Psychiatry* 2001;62 Suppl 17:16–22.

5. Cottler LB, Nishith P, Compton WM 3rd. Gender differences in risk factors for trauma exposure and post-traumatic stress disorder among inner-city drug abusers in and out of treatment. *Comprehensive Psychiatry* 2001;42:111–7.

6. Hutton, HE, Treisman GJ, Hunt WR, Fishman M, Kendig N, Swetz A, Lyketsos CG. HIV risk behaviors and their relationship to posttraumatic stress disorder among women prisoners. *Psychiatric Services* 2001;52:508–13.

7. Kessler RC, Sonega A, Bromer E. Posttraumatic stress disorder in the national comorbidity survey. *Archives of General Psychiatry* 1995;52:1048–60.

8. Najavits LM, Weiss RD, Shaw SR. The link between substance abuse and posttraumatic stress disorder in women. *American Journal of Addictions* 1997;6:274–83.

9. Robins LH, Regier DA (eds). *Psychiatric Disorders in America: The Epidemiological Catchment Area Study.* New York: Free Press, 1991.

10. Curtis JR, Wenrich MD, Carline JD, Shannon SE, Ambrozy DM, Ramsey PG. "Choice" in end-of-life decision making: researching fact or fiction? *Gerontologist* 2002 Oct.;42 Spec No 3:114–28.

11. Sowell RL, Phillips KD, Grier J. Restructuring life to face the future: the perspective of men after a positive response to protease inhibitor therapy. *AIDS Patient Care STDS* 1998 Jan.;12(1):33–42.

Chapter *8:* Special Problems: Hepatitis C and Adherence

1. National Institutes of Health. Management of hepatitis C. Consensus Development Conference Statement. June 10–12, 2002; 19.

2. McDermott BE, Sautter FJ, Winstead DK, Quirk T. Diagnosis, health beliefs, and risk of HIV infection in psychiatric patients. *Hospital and Community Psychiatry* 1994;45: 580–5.

3. Yates WR, Gleason O. Hepatitis C and depression. *Depression and Anxiety* 1998;7: 188–93.

4. Johnson ME, Fisher DG, Fenaughty A, Theno SA. Hepatitis C virus and depression in drug users. *American Journal of Gastroenterology* 1998;93:785–9.

5. Miyaoka H, Otsubo T, Kamijima K, Ishii M, Onuki M, Mitamura K. Depression from interferon therapy in patients with hepatitis C. *American Journal of Psychiatry* 1999;156:1120.

6. Musselman DL, Lawson DH, Gumnick JF, Manatunga AK, Penna S, Goodkin RS, Greiner K, Nemeroff CB, Miller AH. Paroxetine for the prevention of depression induced by interferon alfa. *New England Journal of Medicine* 2001;344:961–6.

7. Larder BA, Darby G, Richman DD. HIV with reduced sensitivity to zidovudine (AZT) isolated during prolonged therapy. *Science* 1989;243:1731–4.

8. Kirkland LR, Fischl MA, Tashima KT, Paar D, Gensler T, Graham NM, Gao H, Rosenzweig JR, McClernon DR, Pittman G, Hessenthaler SM, Hernandez JE; The NZTA4007 Study Team. Response to lamivudine-zidovudine plus abacavir twice daily in antiretroviral-naive, incarcerated patients with HIV infection taking directly observed treatment. *Clinical Infectious Diseases* 2002 Feb. 15; 34(4):511–18.

9. Moreno A, Perez-Elias MJ, Casado JL, Munoz V, Antela A, Dronda F, Navas E, Fortun J, Quereda C, Moreno S. Effectiveness and pitfalls of initial highly active antiretroviral therapy in HIV-infected patients in routine clinical practice. *Antiviral Therapy* 2000 Dec.;5(4):243–8.

10. Paterson DL, Swindells S, Mohr J, Brester M, Vergis EN, Squier C, Wagener MM, Singh N. Adherence to protease inhibitor therapy and outcomes in patients with HIV infection. *Annals of Internal Medicine* 2000;133:21–30.

11. Lee R, Monteiro EF. Third regional audit of antiretroviral prescribing in HIV patients. *International Journal of Studies in AIDS* 2003 Jan.;14(1):58–60.

12. Kleeberger CA, Phair JP, Strathdee SA, Detels R, Kingsley L, Jacobson LP. Determinants of heterogeneous adherence to HIV-antiretroviral therapies in the Multicenter AIDS Cohort Study. *Journal of Acquired Immune Deficiency Syndromes* 2001 Jan.; 126(1):82–92.

13. Gifford AL, Bormann JE, Shively MJ, Wright BC, Richman DD, Bozzette SA. Predictors of self-reported adherence and plasma HIV concentrations in patients on multidrug antiretroviral regimens. *Journal of Acquired Immune Deficiency Syndromes* 2000 Apr. 15;23(5):386–95.

14. Lucas GM, Chaisson RE, Moore RD. Highly active antiretroviral therapy in a large urban clinic: risk factors for virologic failure and adverse drug reactions. *Annals of Internal Medicine* 1999 July 20;131(2):81–7.

15. Altice FL, Mostashari F, Friedland GH. Trust and the acceptance of and adherence to antiretroviral therapy. *Journal of Acquired Immune Deficiency Syndromes* 2001 Sept. 1; 28(1):47–58.

16. Stone VE, Clarke J, Lovell J, Steger KA, Hirschhorn LR, Boswell S, Monroe AD, Stein MD, Tyree TJ, Mayer KH. HIV/AIDS patients' perspectives on adhering to regimens containing protease inhibitors. *Journal of General Internal Medicine* 1998 Sept.; 13(9):586–93.

17. Singh N, Squier C, Sivek C, Wagener M, Nguyen MH, Yu VL. Determinants of compliance with antiretroviral therapy in patients with human immunodeficiency virus: prospective assessment with implications for enhancing compliance. *AIDS Care* 1996;8: 261–9.

18. Fairfield KM, Libman H, Davis RB, Eisenberg DM. Delays in protease inhibitor use in clinical practice. *Journal of General Internal Medicine* 1999;14:395–401.

19. Ickovics JR, Hamburger ME, Vlahov D, Schoenbaum EE, Schuman P, Boland RJ, Moore J; HIV Epidemiology Research Study Group. Mortality, CD4 cell count decline, and depressive symptoms among HIV-seropositive women: Longitudinal analysis from the HIV Epidemiology Research Study. *JAMA* 2001;285:1466–74.

20. Carrieri MP, Chesney MA, Spire B, Loundou A, Sobel A, Lepeu G, Moatti JP. Failure to maintain adherence to HAART in a cohort of French HIV-positive injecting drug users. *International Journal of Behavioral Medicine* 2003;10(1):1–14.

21. Gordillo V, del Amo J, Soriano V, Gonzalez-Lahoz J. Sociodemographic and psychological variables influencing adherence to antiretroviral therapy. *AIDS* 1999 Sept. 10; 13(13):1763–9.

22. Wilson TE, Ickovics JR, Fernandez MI, Koenig LJ, Walter E. Self-reported zidovudine adherence among pregnant women with human immunodeficiency virus infection in four US states. *American Journal of Obstetrics and Gynecology* 2001 May; 184(6): 1235–40.

Chapter *9:* How to Fight AIDS

1. Atkinson S, Bihari D, Smithies M, Daly K, Mason R, McColl I. Identification of futility in intensive care. *Lancet* 1994;344:203–6.

Index